Beyond Activities

Learning Experiences to Support the National Physical Education Standards

S E C O N D A R Y

Susan P. Kogut, Editor

National Association for Sport and Physical Education

An Association of the
**American Alliance for Health, Physical Education,
Recreation and Dance**

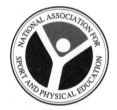

Address orders to: AAHPERD Publications, P.O. Box 385, Oxon Hill, MD 20750-0385, call 1-800-321-0789, or order on line at www.aahperd.org/naspe.
Order Stock No. 304-10268.

Printed in the United States of America.

ISBN 0-88314-901-X

Table of Contents

Preface iv

Introduction v

National Content Standards
For Physical Education vi

Grades 6-8

Striking Volcano 1
Basketball Jam Dance 9
Dances for Groups of 4 17
Racetrack Physical Activity Routine 21
Learning Fitness Concepts with Movement 25
Understanding Intensity and Perceived Exertion 37
Strike and Volley 41
Beef Basketball 45
The Heart Stock Market 49
Fitness Choreography 55

Grades 8-12

Tinikling and Jump Bands 59
Track & Field Fitness Routine 63
Students Creatively Leading Aerobics 73
Discovering Agility in Soccer 81
Jump Rope School 85
Cooperative Beating Hearts 89
Scramble Fitness Dice 93
Changing Intensity Levels to Fit Your Fitness Program 99
Score on Skill 101
Archery Made Simple, and Maybe Golf? 105

Resources 109

Preface

NASPE has been engaged since 1995 in promoting and supporting Moving Into the Future: National Standards for Physical Education (1995). Now, in 2003, over 25,000 copies have been distributed and most states have adopted these standards or aligned program frameworks with them to varying degrees. For the first time, there is a written profession-wide statement of what a student should know and be able to do to be a physically educated person.

In addition to the standards, NASPE has also developed statements of appropriate practice describing supportive teaching strategies and behaviors to support student learning in physical education at each educational level. For many years, NASPE has recommended specific "opportunity-to-learn" or program supports for physical education including time, qualified teachers, and class size, among many others. In the last five years, NASPE has published thirteen titles in the Assessment Series for physical education to help teachers with techniques to assess student achievement of the standards. All of these activities have provided assistance to school districts and teachers as they work to provide quality physical education programs.

The remaining variable in providing a quality physical education program is the learning experiences that teachers use or design to help students learn and practice the knowledge and skills reflected in the standards. The elementary and secondary volumes of *Beyond Activities: Learning Experiences to Support the National Physical Education Standards* provide tried and true activities used by accomplished and recognized teachers to implement standards-based quality physical education.

Susan Kogut, a National Teacher of the Year, has selected and edited the activities submitted in response to a solicitation to all Teachers of the Year as well as physical education teachers who have been certified as "accomplished teachers" by the National Board for Professional Teaching Standards. The activities that have been selected represent the "best from the best" suggestions for learning experiences related to the national standards. However, they are only examples that we hope will stimulate the design of many more high quality learning experiences as teachers use them, adapt them and extend them to meet the needs of their own students.

I would like to acknowledge each and every contributor for helping to improve all physical education by sharing their expertise with more than "just activities."

Judith C. Young, Ph.D.
Executive Director
National Association for Sport and Physical Education

Introduction

Activities are the core of a physical education program. Specific activities, however, are the means to the end and not the purpose of the lesson. Lesson plans that include activities with a clear learning purpose are a required element in an appropriate physical education program that also supports the national standards.

Beyond Activities is a collection of instructionally and developmentally appropriate learning experiences, each with a specific learning focus. The purpose of this publication is to demonstrate how learning experiences that reflect NASPE's national content standards can be implemented effectively. The examples that have been used were selected from materials submitted by NASPE Teachers of the Year and teachers certified by the National Board for Professional Teaching Standards who have used the described lessons in actual classroom settings.

The national standards that are supported are stated specifically for each learning experience, along with a simple statement of what the students should learn from this experience. Each experience suggests a teaching strategy, indicating how the skill could be delivered, along with instructional cues that will guide student performance. Assessment will be facilitated by the feedback provided by these instructional cues.

Each learning experience provides several practice activities, giving the students many opportunities to practice the skills involved in order to increase the potential for success. Using a progression of tasks from simple to more complex and incorporating different kinds of equipment provide the necessary variation to assure success and challenge for students of all skill levels. A culminating activity will allow the learned skill to be used in a fun, practical and challenging way. This is also the opportunity for the isolated skill or concept to be integrated with prior learning and provides the teacher with an opportunity to observe another dimension of student understanding and skill acquisition.

An assessment strategy is identified for each activity, because ongoing assessment is a critical and integral part of the teaching process. Practical, ready-to-use assessments with reproducible score sheets and task sheets are included with each of the learning experiences to help teachers provide a fully comprehensive learning process. The assessment suggestions will facilitate student learning, guide teacher feedback, provide greater understanding of the skill or concept and allow documentation of student progress.

In this book, the NASPE Teachers of the year and Board certified teachers share practical learning experiences. There is no attempt to be exhaustive in representing all NASPE standards and benchmarks for all grades. However, it is hoped that these practical learning experiences will be useful, adaptable, and serve as a model to stimulate new ideas. We hope that this teacher resource will lead to reflection about student learning in relation to the national standards for physical education and will lead to new teacher-generated strategies and learning activities to enhance physical education programs. Quality physical education (QPE) consists of providing students with:*

◆ Opportunity to learn

◆ Important content

◆ Excellent and appropriate instructional practice

The lessons included in this book reflect all of these qualities, and therefore represent model blueprints for quality physical education!

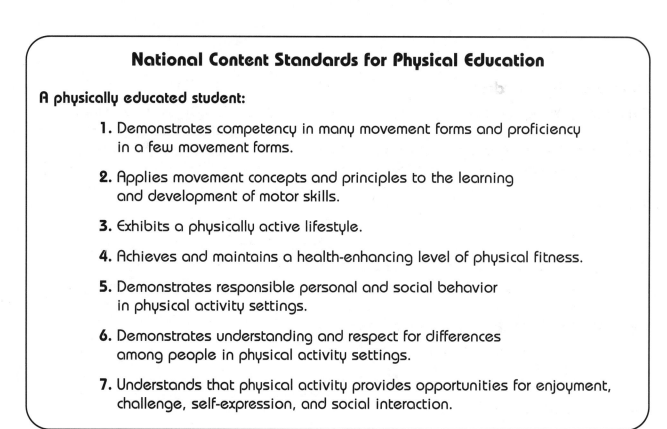

National Content Standards for Physical Education

A physically educated student:

1. Demonstrates competency in many movement forms and proficiency in a few movement forms.

2. Applies movement concepts and principles to the learning and development of motor skills.

3. Exhibits a physically active lifestyle.

4. Achieves and maintains a health-enhancing level of physical fitness.

5. Demonstrates responsible personal and social behavior in physical activity settings.

6. Demonstrates understanding and respect for differences among people in physical activity settings.

7. Understands that physical activity provides opportunities for enjoyment, challenge, self-expression, and social interaction.

*A complete listing of the NASPE publications containing these guidelines and standards can be found in Resources at the end of this book.

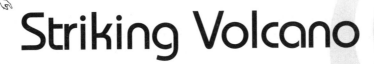

Striking Volcano

Nancy J. Markos
2002 National Elementary School Teacher of the Year
Broadus Wood Elementary School—Earlysville, VA

Pam Walker
1996 Virginia Elementary School Teacher of the Year
Red Hill Elementary School—North Garden, VA

Stephanie Almquist
Churchill Road Elementary School—Fairfax County, VA

National Standards:

Standard 1: Demonstrates competency in the movement form of underhand striking.

Standard 5: Demonstrates responsible social behavior while participating in practice activities and in peer assessment.

Students Will Learn:

The underhand strike

Teaching Strategy:

Interactive/practice

How Students Will Be Organized:

The students will be in small practice groups based on the different needs of the various activities.

Cues For Instruction:

Ready: Face in the direction of the hit, feet shoulder width apart, eyes looking forward, ball held in past the front midline of the body at waist level.

Arm Back: Pull striking arm back past the side midline of the body to waist level.

Step and Hit: Step with foot on nonstriking side while heel of striking hand contacts the underside of the ball in front of the body at waist level or below.

Follow Through: Striking hand continues in the direction of the ball but does not go beyond the height of the shoulder.

Other Cue Sets—choose cues that mean something to your students:
Ready, Step, Hit.
Hold it, Low, Step, Hit.
Start, Extend, Step and Swing, Follow through.

Practice Activities:

Locomotor—Sneak Attack
Objective: To give students individual practice on the underhand strike. Also to give teachers a chance to quickly assess and help children on the skill's different components.
Equipment: Space
Directions: Review the components of the underhand strike. Tell the students what locomotor skill to use. Have the students move around in general space using the selected locomotor skill; then the teacher will call out different components of the underhand strike. Students will stop, show the teacher the component, and then move again. Teachers can continually change the different locomotor skills.

Balloon Strike
Objective: To give students individual practice with the underhand strike.
Equipment: One balloon for each student
Directions: Review the components of the underhand strike. Have the students get into their own space and practice hitting their balloon using the underhand strike. Have them hit the balloon and then run to catch it before it hits the ground. Repeat as many times as needed. Have the students hit the balloon and catch it as many times as they can in one minute, then have them repeat the process to see if they can do better.

Wall Targets With Varying Distances
Objective: To give students individual practice at hitting targets using the underhand strike.
Equipment: One ball per student (gator ball, beach ball, etc.), one to three targets per student, tape, space with four walls.
Directions: Before the students arrive, mark off a practice area for each child. Each practice area needs to have one to three targets on the wall and the floor needs to have three pieces of tape on it, one at the back of the area, the other two progressively closer to the wall. Have students go to their practice areas and stand on the tape closest to the wall. Using the assigned ball, students try to hit all of the targets. When they succeed, they can move to the second closest piece of tape, and so on. They are finished when they hit all the targets from all three pieces of tape.

Hitting Beach Balls To Partner
Objective: To give students the opportunity to practice the underhand strike with a partner.
Equipment: One beach ball for every two students.

Directions: Review the components of the underhand strike with students. Have one student use the underhand strike to get the beach ball to the other student so that it can be caught. The partner returns the ball the same way, using the underhand strike. If partners accomplish this, have them take one step back and try again. If they do not make it, have them stay where they are or take one step forward.

Create A Word

Objective: To give students the opportunity to practice the underhand strike with a partner. To give students the opportunity to practice the underhand strike while reviewing vocabulary words.

Equipment: Two sets of letters of the alphabet (with extra commonly used letters), vocabulary words, one ball for every two students (beach ball or gator ball).

Directions: Before students arrive, randomly post the letters of the alphabet on the wall. Review components of the underhand strike with students. Assign partners and give them one ball and one vocabulary list. Partners are to spell out each word on the vocabulary list by using the underhand strike to hit the letter they need. They look for the letter on the wall, take a predetermined number of steps from the wall, and then perform the underhand strike. Partners keep working on that letter until they can hit the letter. Partners can alternate letters or words.

Wall Ball

Objective: To use small group or partner activities to help work on the underhand strike.

Equipment: One gator ball or playground ball for every two to three players, a lot of wall space.

Directions: Review the components of the underhand strike with students. Put students in-groups of no more than three-students A, B, and C. Student A underhand strikes the ball to Student B, and Student B catches it before it hits the ground. Student B underhand strikes the ball to Student C, Student C catches the ball before it hits the ground. Student C underhand strikes the ball to Student A, Student A catches the ball before it hits the ground. If the ball hits the ground before it is caught, the last person to strike the ball gets a point. Vary the game by changing the number of times the ball is allowed to bounce before it is caught, depending on students' ability and age.

Small Court Games

Objectives: To use lead-up games to help students practice using the underhand strike.

Equipment: One folding mat, one ball, and four cones per four students, one poly dot for each student.

Directions: Before students arrive, create small courts for every four students and mark them off with four cones. Then place two poly dots on either side of an accordion mat, which is standing in the middle of each court. Review the components of the underhand strike with students. Assign each student to a poly dot, which automatically puts each student on a team. The first person with the ball underhand strikes it to the other side. The other side has to catch the ball without letting it hit the ground. Players may not step off the poly dot to catch the ball. If the ball hits the ground, the team that struck the ball gains one point. If the ball is caught or goes out of bounds, the catching team gains a point. The catching team now becomes the striking team. It is important to make sure the teams rotate strikers. To vary the game, students can come off the poly dots a certain number of steps. Another way to vary the game is to have students continue to volley the ball over the mat.

Switcharoo

Objective: To use large group activities to work on the underhand strike.

Equipment: Several gator balls and/or beach balls, a field or preferably a gymnasium with markers to split it in half.

Directions: Review the underhand strike with students. Split the class in half so that there is half a class on either side of the dividing line. This game is played similarly to the game "get rid of the garbage." The object of the game is to get rid of all the balls on your side of the gymnasium by hitting the ball to the other side. However, players do not want opposing teammates to catch the hit ball. Students are to underhand strike any ball on their side of the gym (students may be in control of only one ball at a time) to the other side. If the other team catches the ball, the striker needs to switch to the other side.

Culminating Activity:

Volcano

Objective: To use a large group activity to practice the underhand strike. To use the underhand strike and work on math skills.

Equipment: Three accordion mats, several poly dots, several gator balls or beach balls

Directions: Stand the accordion mats next to each other in the shape of a circle, which makes the volcano. Scatter poly dots around the outside of the volcano. Assign a point value to the poly dots (i.e., red=1, purple=2). Select a few students to stand inside the volcano. The other students get a ball, and go stand on a poly dot and underhand strike the ball into the volcano. If they are successful they earn the number of points the poly dot is worth. The students in the center throw out any ball that lands in the middle. Students on the outside of the volcano keep track of their points and keep hitting balls into the volcano until the time is up. When the time is up, the class adds up all the points each student gained to come up with a class score. Now, select new students to be in the center and have the class try to break its record.

To vary the game and to keep students honest, pair up the strikers. That way they can check each other's math and make sure they are not giving themselves too many points.

Assessment:

Partner check sheet—partners will observe five trials and mark check sheet accordingly.

Teacher check sheet—To be completed as the students are involved in the practice activities. Each student will have many opportunities to perform the correct instructional cues.

Teacher Assessment Sheet

Class: _____ Objective: _____ Pre: _____
Post: _____

Student	Ready Position	Arm Back	Step and Hit	Follow Through	Comments

Partner Skill Check

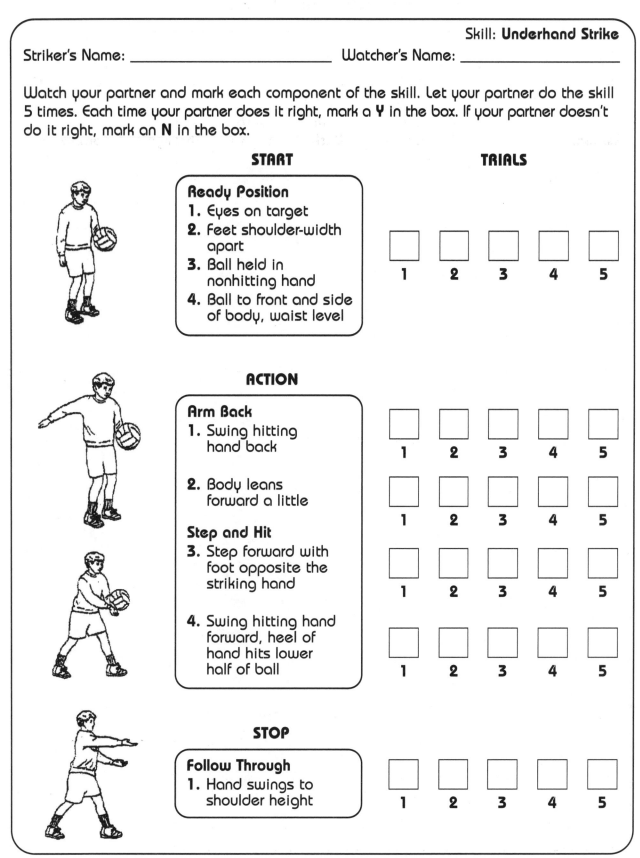

Skill: **Underhand Strike**

Striker's Name: _____ Watcher's Name: _____

Watch your partner and mark each component of the skill. Let your partner do the skill 5 times. Each time your partner does it right, mark a **Y** in the box. If your partner doesn't do it right, mark an **N** in the box.

START

TRIALS

Ready Position
1. Eyes on target
2. Feet shoulder-width apart
3. Ball held in nonhitting hand
4. Ball to front and side of body, waist level

☐ ☐ ☐ ☐ ☐
1 2 3 4 5

ACTION

Arm Back
1. Swing hitting hand back

☐ ☐ ☐ ☐ ☐
1 2 3 4 5

2. Body leans forward a little

☐ ☐ ☐ ☐ ☐
1 2 3 4 5

Step and Hit
3. Step forward with foot opposite the striking hand

☐ ☐ ☐ ☐ ☐
1 2 3 4 5

4. Swing hitting hand forward, heel of hand hits lower half of ball

☐ ☐ ☐ ☐ ☐
1 2 3 4 5

STOP

Follow Through
1. Hand swings to shoulder height

☐ ☐ ☐ ☐ ☐
1 2 3 4 5

Beyond Activities

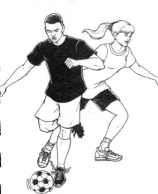

Basketball Jam Dance

Melanie Champion
2001 National Middle School Teacher of the Year
South Brunswick Middle School—Southport, NC

National Standards:

Standard 1: Demonstrate competency in movement patterns and specific dance steps.

Standard 5: Student will work with a partner, and in a group, to learn, practice, and assess the dance sequences.

Students Will Learn:

Dance steps, basketball skills, and social responsibility.

Teaching Strategy:

Task style, guided discovery

How Students Will Be Organized:

Small groups

Cues for Instruction:

The feedback relating to the dance steps during the dance practice and then those relating to ball handling when that skill is added. The students follow the cues on the instruction sheet and help each other in the group. Students must be able to perform one part before going on to the next.

Practice Activities:

- ◆ The line dance is broken down into 4-6 parts and explained on task cards, which are lettered in order of occurrence (abcd).
- ◆ The groups each learn and practice the dance without the basketballs and check each other for understanding.
- ◆ Each group must master each part and then put the entire dance together to music.

Culminating Activity: The Jam

Add basketballs to the dance and have students perform the entire dance together.

Assessment:

The task sheet for self-, teacher and peer assessment is included along with the rubric levels.

The S.B.M.S. Basketball Jam—Space Jam—By Quad City

- Finger touches with a basketball (or a ball that bounces) for eight counts in front of the waist while alternating right, left, right, left heel raises.
- Finger touches with a basketball (or a ball that bounces) for eight counts above the head while alternating right, left, right, left, heel raises.
- Side Step out with the right foot to the side, close with the left foot, repeat and power dribble once on the last step. Side Step out with the left foot to the side, close with the right, repeat and power dribble once on the last step. **REPEAT.**
- Grapevine right and pump fake shot with your ball on the last step (step with right foot out to side, behind the right foot with the left foot, out to the side with the right and together with the left foot). Repeat to the left with the grapevine and pump fake shot with your ball on the last step. Repeat grapevine right and left with shot.
- Walk forward four steps starting with your right foot and slam-dunk the ball with both hands on the fourth step.
- Walk backward four steps starting with your left foot and slam-dunk the ball backwards with both hands on the fourth step.
- Repeat walking forward and backward with the slam-dunks.
- Using your left foot as a pivot foot, step forward diagonally with your right foot and then back diagonally with your right foot and repeat forward and back holding the ball with both hands.
- Feet shoulder width apart, holding the ball with both hands, do ball fakes starting to the left- return to middle, right- return to middle, left- return to middle, and right- return to middle.
- Repeat Dance.

Name: _____ Grade: _____

Music: "Space Jam" by Quad City DJs

Do each step until you feel you have accomplished that step. Upon completion, check the space provided beside the step and advance to the next step. **Do not advance until you know the steps well enough to do it without looking at the directions.**

1. _____ For the first 8 counts do finger touches with a basketball (or a ball that bounces) in front of the waist while alternating right, left, right, left heel raises.

2. _____ Finger touches with a basketball (or a ball that bounces) above the head while alternating right, left, right, left heel raises for the next 8 counts.

3. _____ Side step out with right foot to the side, close with left foot and repeat, power dribbling once on the last step. Side step out with the left foot to the side, close with right foot and repeat, power dribbling once on the last step.
Repeat

4. _____ Grapevine right and pump fake shot with your ball on last step. (Grapevine: step with right foot out to side, behind the right foot with the left foot, out to the side with the right and together with the left foot.) Repeat to the left with the grapevine and pump fake shot with your ball on the last step.
Repeat grapevine right and left with shot.

5. _____ Walk forward four steps starting with right foot and slam-dunk ball with both hands on the fourth step. Walk backward four steps starting with left foot and slam-dunk backward with both hands on the fourth step.
Repeat walking forward and backward with slam-dunks.

6. _____ For 8 counts, holding the ball with both hands and using your left foot as a pivot foot, step forward diagonally with right foot and then back diagonally with your right foot and repeat forward and back.

7. _____ Place feet shoulder width apart, holding the ball with both hands. For 8 counts do ball fakes starting to the left, return to middle, right, return to middle, left, return to middle, and right, return to middle.

8. _____ Practice all steps together in order several times until you have it!

9. _____ Check if you know the "Space Jam" dance!

Variation: A slower version can be done to "The Winner" by Coolio on the Space Jam CD.

Line Dance Rubric Pattern—Level 1

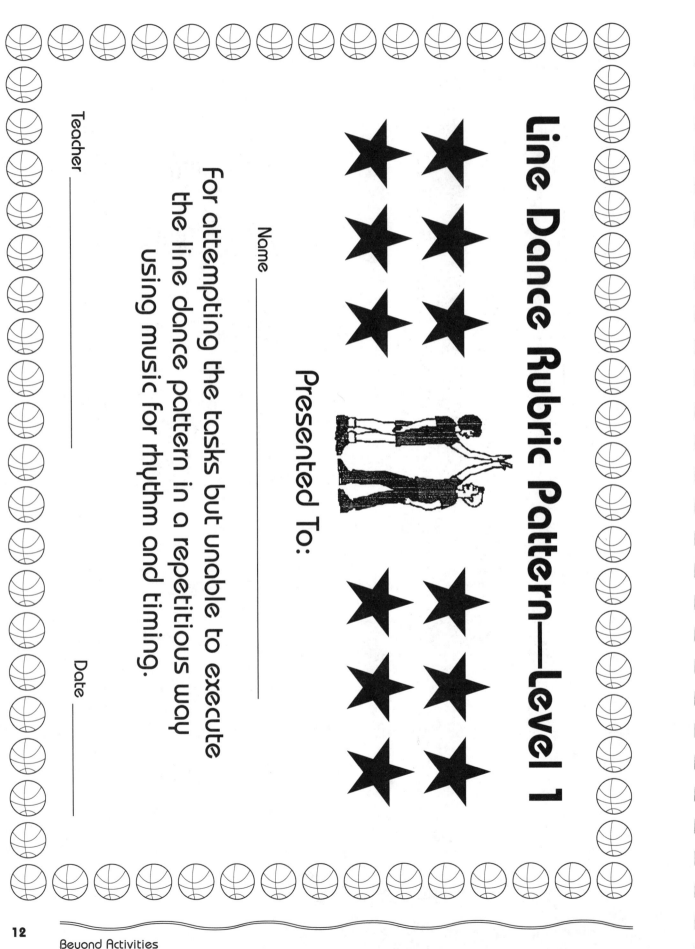

Presented To:

Name _____

For attempting the tasks but unable to execute the line dance pattern in a repetitious way using music for rhythm and timing.

Teacher _____

Date _____

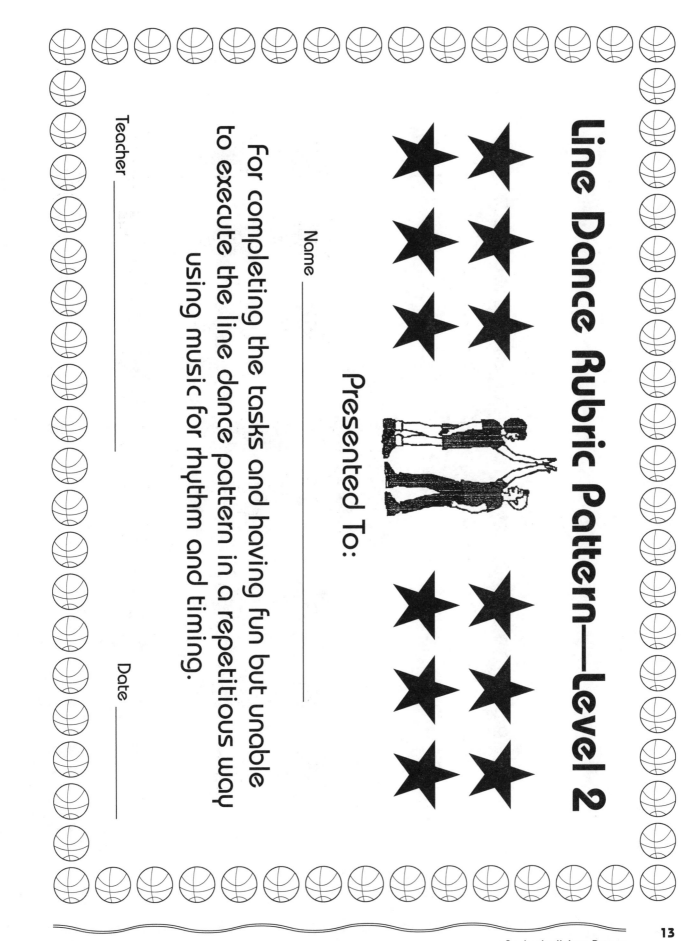

Line Dance Rubric Pattern—Level 2

Presented To:

Name _____

For completing the tasks and having fun but unable to execute the line dance pattern in a repetitious way using music for rhythm and timing.

Teacher _____

Date _____

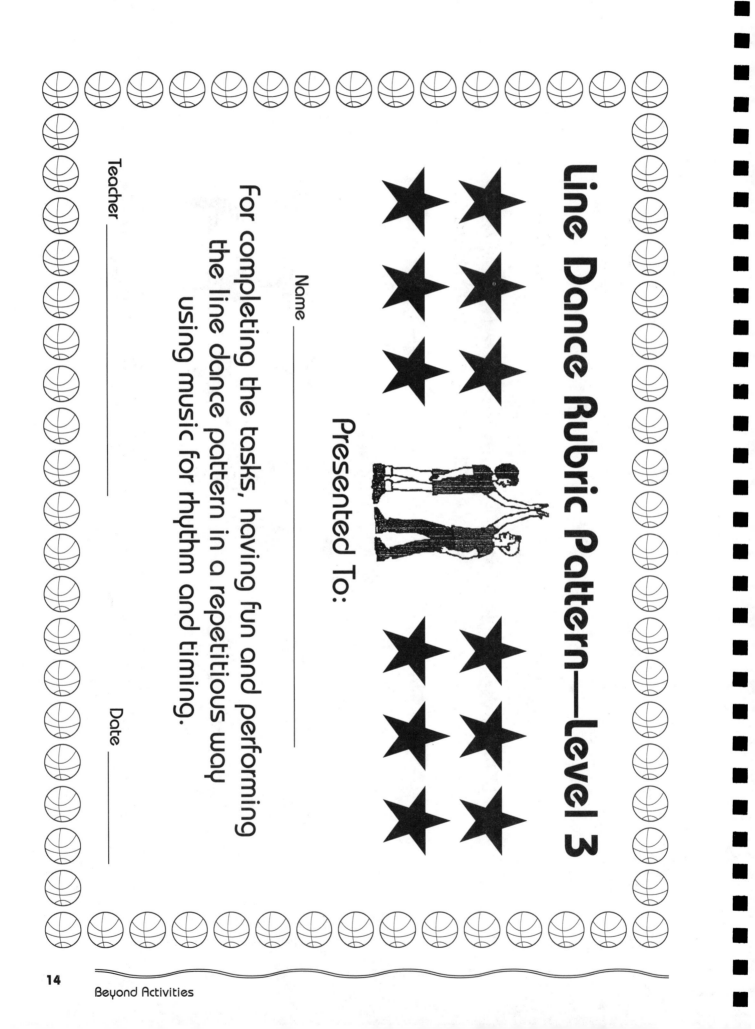

Line Dance Rubric Pattern—Level 3

Presented To:

_____
Name

For completing the tasks, having fun and performing the line dance pattern in a repetitious way using music for rhythm and timing.

Teacher _____

Date _____

Line Dance Rubric Pattern—Level 4

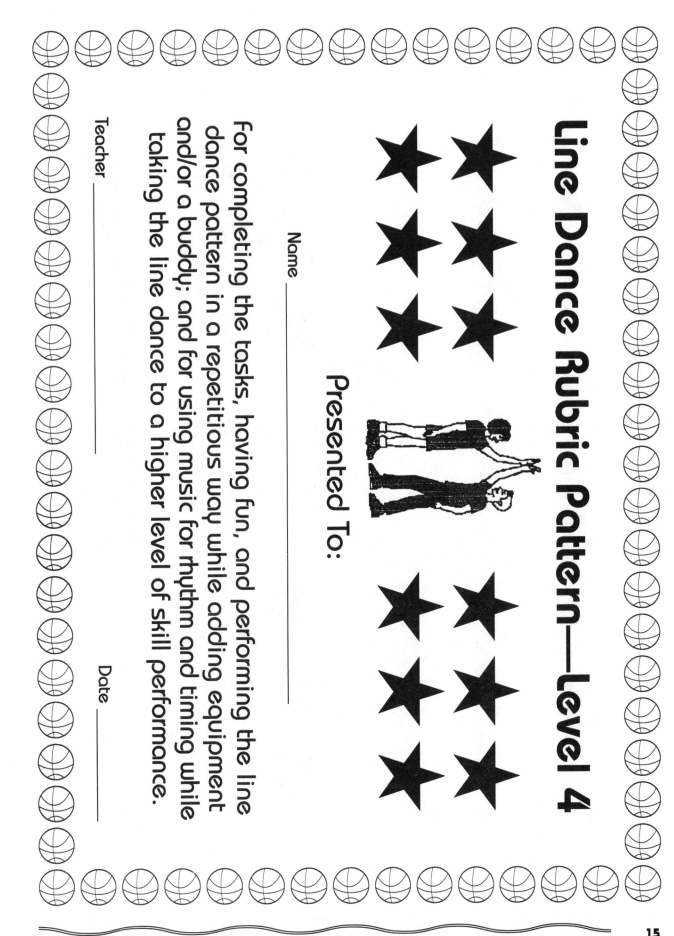

Presented To:

Name _____

For completing the tasks, having fun, and performing the line dance pattern in a repetitious way while adding equipment and/or a buddy; and for using music for rhythm and timing while taking the line dance to a higher level of skill performance.

Teacher _____

Date _____

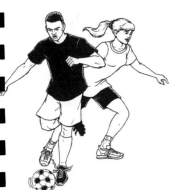

Dances for Groups of 4

Charlene A. Darst
2001 National Elementary School Teacher of the Year
Whitman Elementary School—Mesa, AZ

Paul W. Darst
Arizona State University—Tempe, AZ

National Standards:

Standard 1: Competency is demonstrated in the learner's ability to perform each of the moves correctly and in rhythm to the music.

Standard 5: Success of the group's ability to perform the dances is dependent on each other.

Students Will Learn:

To perform a sequence of specific square dance moves rhythmically to the music.

Teaching Strategy:

Jig saw

How Students Will Be Organized:

Students will work in groups of four. Four stations will be set up, one in each corner of the gymnasium. Digital camera pictures work wonderfully to provide a visual for your students. A different skill will be listed on each station sign:
- do-si-do,
- right-hand and left-hand star,
- elbow swing with partner, and with corner and allemande left with corner, and
- circle left and right with your group of four.

One person from each group will be sent to a different station to learn that individual skill. All four will come back together and be responsible for teaching each person in their original group of four the new dance skill that they learned.

Students will learn all individual parts without music, use them with teacher-directed cues without music and then perform them to the music with teacher cues.

The teacher can gradually speed up the cues to prepare the students for faster moving music.

Cues For Instruction:

Do-si-do: pass right shoulder to partner as you walk forward, then pass left shoulders as you walk backwards, do not turn around

Elbow swing: rest elbow on waist and circle around once, under control

Right-hand star: join right hands in the center, walk clockwise

Left-hand star: join left hands in the center, walk counter clockwise

Circle the ring: all join hands and circle clockwise or counter clockwise

Allemande left with your corner: turn and face your corner, join left hands, turn once around to come back to your partner

Practice Activities:

Three dances requiring four people per group will be the focus of this Rhythms lesson. *Four People Square Dance* (Joyce Ellis, Central District Middle School Teacher of the Year 2001—AAHPERD Conference, San Diego), *Big Sombrero Mixer* and *Oh Johnny, Oh Johnny, Oh* (Dynamic Physical Education for Elementary School Students—Pangrazi, 13th edition).

1. *Four People Square Dance*
Formation—Groups of 4, each with a partner
Skills—do-si-do, elbow swing,
Music—Grandma's Feather Bed from John Denver's Greatest Hits, Vol. 2
- Circle left for 8 cts.
- Walk into the center for 4 cts. and back out for 4 cts.
- Circle right for 8 cts.
- Walk into the center for 4 cts. and back out for 4 cts.
- Do-si-do your partner for 8 cts.
- Do-si-do your corner for 8 cts.
- Swing your partner for 8 cts.
- Swing your corner for 8 cts.
- Repeat the dance

2. *Oh Johnny, Oh Johnny, Oh*
Skills—do-si-do, elbow swing, allemande left, promenade
Formation—groups of four each with a partner
Music—traditional—WWCD-05114; WWC-57
Wagon Wheel Records
17151 Corbina Lane #212
Huntington Beach, CA 92649
(714) 846-8169

- ◆ All join hands and circle the ring for 8 cts.
- ◆ Stop where you are give your partner a swing (Swing your partner) for 4 cts.
- ◆ Swing the little girl behind you (swing corner) for 4 cts.
- ◆ Now swing your own (swing partner) for 4 cts.
- ◆ Allemande left with the corner gal (allemande left with your corner) for 4 cts.
- ◆ You do-si-do with your own (do si do your partner) for 4 cts.
- ◆ Then you all promenade
- ◆ With your sweet corner maid (promenade with your corner—walk around the circle)
- ◆ Singing Oh Johnny, Oh Johnny, Oh!
- ◆ Repeat the sequence with your new partner

3. *Big Sombrero Mixer*
Skills—do-si-do, rt. hand and lft. hand star, elbow swing
Formation—2 sets of partners form a square
Music—Marc Anthony—I Need to Know
Begin actions when the words to the song begin
- ◆ 8 counts: Walk in circle to the left with group of four
- ◆ 8 counts: Walk in circle to the right with group of four
- ◆ 8 counts: Do-si-do with partner
- ◆ 8 counts: Do-si-do with corner
- ◆ 8 counts: All four right hand star
- ◆ 8 counts: All four left hand star
- ◆ 8 counts: Right elbow swing with partner
- ◆ 8 counts: One couple passes through right shoulders to right shoulders and walk on to the next couple to make a new set of four

Culminating Activity:

Each class will select one of the four dances to perform for their teacher at the conclusion of the class. Most skills taught in one dance will be used in another dance. Rhythms units should be interspersed throughout the year as opposed to doing all your rhythms within one unit. The skills learned in this lesson will carry over into the next one-week unit of rhythms.

Assessment:

The teacher is continually scanning the class and moving throughout the area, as calls are being given, to make sure that all learners are actively involved and are successful in performing each of the individual moves. A checklist will be used to evaluate each skill as it is being taught in the jig saw.

Simple Checklist for Four Person Dances

Name _____ Class _____ Score _____

Place a check beside each cue that is demonstrated correctly.

Do-Si-Do

1. Pass right shoulders   _____
2. Pass left shoulders   _____
3. Does not turn around   _____

Elbow Swing

1. Rests right elbows on waist   _____
2. Turn once around   _____
3. Turn is under control   _____

Allemande Left

1. Left hands are quickly joined   _____
2. Turn around to face opposite direction   _____
3. Pass left shoulders and return back to partner   _____

Star Formation

1. Right hands raised quickly   _____
2. Turn is in clockwise direction   _____
3. Repeat quickly with left hands
   in a counterclockwise direction   _____

Circle with Group

1. Hands are joined quickly   _____
2. Circle to the left 8 counts under control   _____
3. Circle to the right 8 counts under control   _____

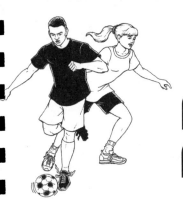

Racetrack Physical Activity Routine

Charlene A. Darst
2001 National Elementary School Teacher of the Year
Whitman Elementary School—Mesa, AZ

Paul W. Darst
Arizona State University—Tempe, AZ

National Standards:

Standard 3: Students are physically active in class and are encouraged to use the activities after school and for the rest of their lives.

Standard 4: Students are learning the knowledge and the skill progressions for the components of health related fitness. They learn and practice the balance necessary to enhance their individual levels of fitness.

Students Will Learn:

Students will be learning the principles of warm-up, the components of health related fitness and progressions for upper body strength, abdominal strength, and flexibility.

Teaching Strategy:

The task style with choices for students at the stations.

How Students Will Be Organized:

Station signs will be set up around the perimeter of the teaching area. Students will work with a partner. One person moves around the perimeter of the area (on the racetrack) performing the teacher-specified cardiovascular exercise while the other partner works on a specific strength or flexibility exercise progression from the fitness sign (refer to Progressive Fitness Challenges).

Cues for Instruction:

Students will have many opportunities to make activity choices in this routine. Choices will be provided to develop cardiovascular fitness, flexibility, abdominal strength, and upper body strength. Students will be directed to hold their stretches for a minimum of 10 seconds.

Students should be encouraged to make their own choices so that they can be successful and challenged at each station.

Reinforcement should be provided for correct stretching positions and for holding the stretch for 10 counts.

Practice Activities:

Refer to attached Racetrack Fitness sign, which can be copied for personal use.

Culminating Activity:

This fitness activity routine in itself is a culminating activity. Students must have previous knowledge of activity choices in order to successfully participate in this routine. This is an excellent fitness choice for teaching the exercise progressions early in the year, and also as a challenge for later in the year.

Assessment:

At the conclusion of class, students will be asked to show four different exercise progressions for each of the following fitness components: flexibility, upper body strength, and abdominal strength. Teachers can ask students, "With a show of fingers, show how long you will hold each stretch?"

Students need to list four different cardiovascular movements that were performed around the perimeter.

Progressive Fitness Challenges

Developmental Level I (K-2)

Arm-Shoulder Girdle Lead-ups or Upper Body Strength

Bridge position
- Wave an arm and or leg at a friend
- Walk to a friend and give them a high five
- Scratch your back
- Take small jumps while keeping your hands on the ground
- Do a series of turnovers

Crab position
- Crab walk
- Shake an arm and or leg
- Walk on two hands and one foot

Push-up position
- Walk your feet up to your hands and back
- Lower one knee. Bend arms and touch nose to the floor—gradually move
- your head farther in front of you
- Perform flat tire push-ups

Abdominal Strength Lead-ups:

Laying in a *supine* position without the use of arms or hands and the head held off the ground:
- Lift up your head and look at your toes
- Wiggle your toes as you watch
- Lift up your head and wave to a friend
- Lift your heels off the ground about 6 inches and wave them at a friend
- Sit up, any way you can, and touch your toes
- Lower your body slowly to the floor from a sitting position
- Lift your shoulders and feet off the floor at the same time

Developmental Level II (3-4) and Level III (5-6) Variations

Push-up Variations (Upper Body Strength) (color-coded yellow)
- Regular push-ups
- Modified push-ups
- Push-up position arm circles
- Line push-ups
- Shoulder touch push-ups
- Rest at the bottom push-ups
- Push-up turnovers
- Triceps push-ups
- Crab position push-ups
- Bear crawls
- Crab walks

Abdominal Strength Variations (color-coded blue)
- Curl-ups
- Reverse curl-ups
- Leg extensions
- Rhythmic sit-ups
- Partial curl-up and hold
- V-ups
- Crunches
- Knee-to-chest curls

Adapted from Pangrazi, R.P. 2001. <u>Dynamic Physical Education for Elementary School Children</u>, 13th ed. Boston: Allyn & Bacon.

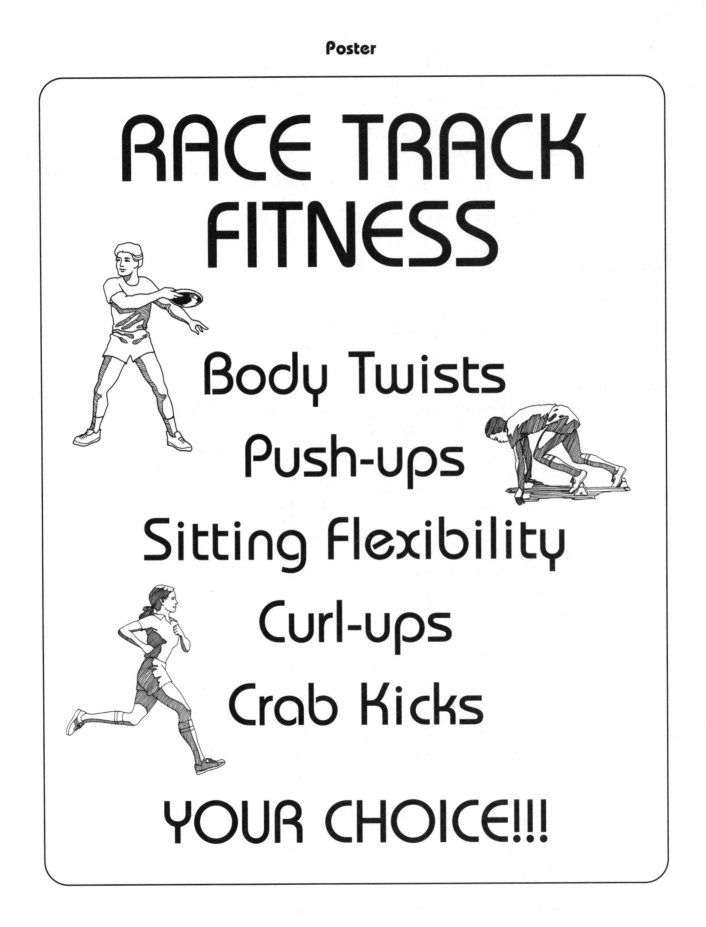

RACE TRACK FITNESS

Body Twists

Push-ups

Sitting Flexibility

Curl-ups

Crab Kicks

YOUR CHOICE!!!

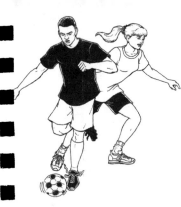

Learning Fitness Concepts with Movement

Grade Level: 6–7

Lois M. Mauch
1997 Central District Middle School Teacher of the Year
Agassiz Middle School—Fargo, ND

National Standards:

Standard 3: Display the ability to apply the principles of fitness to lifestyle.

Standard 5: Understand the importance of self-initiated behavior that promotes personal and group success in fitness education.

Students Will Learn:

- ◆ To use the Fitness Education Pyramid and Heart Rate Monitors
- ◆ To learn the Frequency, Intensity, Time, and Type (F.I.T.T.) principle of fitness
- ◆ To apply the principle to their daily living, to give them a real-life understanding of application.

Teaching Strategy:

Cooperative learning—jig saw

How Students Will Be Organized:

Students will be in groups of five and will have a task form to complete. Each student will visit one of the five stations. Students will report back to their group what they have learned from visiting the station. The group will then complete the task form cooperatively until the entire task form is complete. Additional homework will be given to each student to complete.

Cues for Instruction:

Frequency: The number of times you do the activity

Intensity: How hard you work at the activity, this is usually measured by heart rate or weight in lbs.

Time: How long you work

Type: Aerobic or anaerobic

- ◆ **MHR:** Maximum Heart Rate: Explain that each student has an MHR, which is determined by age. Students subtract their age from 220 to figure out their personal MHR. Then, they can use the Fitness Education Pyramid to determine their target heart rate zones (THZ). By using a heart rate monitor and/or knowing how to take a heart rate, student workouts will be safe.

- ◆ **THZ:** Target Heart Rate Zone: The Target Heart Rate Zone students choose to work out in is personal also. The zone is determined by the student's current lifestyle—someone who works out regularly, might be able to use 70% to 85% of the MHR for the THZ. A student who leads a more sedentary lifestyle may want to use 60% to 75%.

Practice Activities

Fitness Activity—Each group of five will agree on an appropriate fitness warm-up activity. They will self-start and continue until the teacher signals to stop. Learning stations: In groups of five, the students are assigned a color: yellow, green, blue, purple, or red. (If the numbers don't match up just assign two students to the same color) On the signal, students will go to the cone of the color they are and read the information provided about the fitness education pyramid (see attached form). The information is provided on signs that the students can read and tell their group about. Upon returning to their group, they share the information about the F.I.T.T. principles for each color level of the fitness education pyramid and complete the task form as a group. (Students who forget some information, or who do not know task form answers, may return as often as necessary to bring back the information to the group.)

Culminating Activity: Heart Risk Tag

Activity or Game—When groups complete their task forms, students give the forms to the teacher, put on a heart rate monitor, and play Heart Risk Tag or any other tag game. The students should play for about three minutes and then determine the F.I.T.T. principle for that game and which Fitness Education Pyramid Zone they are in.

Heart Risk Tag

Stuff five long socks with old socks and a tie a knot in the ends. Then, use a paint pen to label each sock a health risk factor for heart attacks. Use the yellow sock for *fat* and other colors to represent risks such as *smoking*, *age* (45 and older), *gender* (boys higher than girls), *high blood pressure*, and *stress*. Appoint five people the taggers. They will use the socks and swing below the waist to tag the runners. When someone is tagged, they must stop and wait for another student who is free to come over and stand in front of them. At that time, the free student will say, "I'm a doctor, how will you prevent a heart attack?" The tagged student must answer with a *prevention* such as "I will not smoke," "I will eat right," "I will watch or monitor my blood pressure," "I will exercise daily for 60 minutes." Then they are both free to continue play.

Assessment:

Question/Task, Scoring Rubric

◆ Fill out the task form completely and neatly.

◆ How does your favorite activity apply to the principles of fitness?

◆ Which fitness level applies best to your lifestyle?

◆ Which level applies to your physical fitness level now?

Important Scoring Notes:

◆ Is the form complete?

◆ Did students relate the principles of fitness (F.I.T.T.) to an activity correctly?

◆ Did students pick a fitness education level that best suits their lifestyle?

◆ Did students take task sheet home and apply the information learned to an adult's or sibling's fitness level? (Level 4)

F.I.T.T. Task Form

Students in your group: Class/Period_____

1. _____   6. _____

2. _____   7. _____

3. _____   8. _____

4. _____   9. _____

5. _____   10. _____

Pick the average age of your group:

Age	MHR	Rest HR	40%	50%	70%	80%	85%	95%
11	209	124	135	147	172	184	190	203
12	208	123	134	146	171	183	190	202

If you were 12, what would 85% of your MHR be? _____ Beats Per Minute

If you were 11? _____ Beats Per Minute

Terms you will need to know: The F.I.T.T. Principle

     Frequency: The number of times you do the activity

     Intensity: How hard you work at the activity, usually measured by heart rate or weight in lbs.

     Time: How long you work

     Type: Aerobic or Anaerobic

MHR: Maximum Heart Rate   **THZ:** Target Heart Rate Zone

Weight Management Zone: Yellow

What is the exercise Frequency for the Weight Management Zone? _____

What is the Intensity of the Weight Management Zone? _____

For how much Time? _____

Why would you use this intensity for a workout? _____

What type of activities would qualify for this intensity?
_____

Healthy Heart Zone: Green

What is the exercise Frequency for the Healthy Heart Zone? _____

What is the Intensity of the Healthy Heart Zone? _____

For how much Time? _____

What part of the body does this intensity begin to develop? _____

What type of activities would qualify for this intensity? _____
_____

The Kick-It Zone (Aerobic Zone): Blue

What is the exercise Frequency for the Kick It Zone? _____

What is the Intensity of the Kick It Zone? _____

For how much Time? _____

What two systems of the body begin to develop at this intensity?
1. _____   2. _____

Are the oxygen and carbon dioxide in your muscles being
exchanged during this intensity? _____

What type of activities would qualify for this intensity? _____

The Power Zone (Anaerobic Zone): Purple

What is the exercise Frequency for the Power Zone? _____

What is the Intensity of the Power Zone? _____

For how much Time? _____

This zone is best for metabolizing what?
(It gives you that feeling of stiffness the next day) _____

Are your muscles using oxygen during this intensity? _____

What type of activities would qualify for this intensity? _____

The Red Zone: Red

What is the exercise Frequency for the Red Zone? _____

What is the Intensity of the Red Zone? _____

For how much Time? _____

During this zone you will cross into anaerobic threshold and will be working in oxygen debt? **True** or **False**?

This intensity is only for individuals considered extremely fit. **True** or **False**?

What type of activities would qualify for this intensity? _____

Group Scoring Rubric

Performance Level	Description The group/student has:
4	◆ Completed the task form neatly. ◆ Related an activity to the principles of fitness. ◆ Participated cooperatively.
3	◆ Completed the task form neatly. ◆ Related an activity to the principles of fitness.
2	◆ Completed the task sheet but it is not really neat.
1	◆ Not completed the task sheet.
0	◆ No response or unscoreable

Your Group Score: _____

Comments:

APPLY YOUR OWN LEVEL TO YOUR LIFESTYLE.

◆ On a *separate piece of paper* that you can add to your journal apply your own level to your lifestyle. Remember, the power and red zones are enhancements to the kick-it zone. You want to choose a fitness zone that fits your physical activity goal. Choose from the weight management, healthy heart, or kick-it zones.

What **fitness zone** did you pick? _____

What is the **frequency** used in your zone? _____

What **intensity** would be used for your zone? _____

What is the **time** needed in your zone? _____

Some of the levels overlap in Maximum Heart Rate. Try to understand this material and the feeling of each level. Then, it should be easy to set up your home fitness program.

How would the principles of fitness apply to your favorite activity? (Include the F.I.T.T.)

_____

_____

_____

_____

_____

_____

_____

_____

_____

Extra Credit:

Level Four Assessment: Get a copy of this task sheet and take it home to apply what you have learned to an adult's or an older sibling's fitness level. Figure out their target heart rate zones and the fitness level they should incorporate in their lifestyles. Show your work on the back of this task sheet. Bring it back, signed by the person you shared this with.

Individual Scoring Rubric

Performance Level	Description The student:
4	◆ Completed the task form neatly. ◆ Can relate an activity to the principles of fitness. ◆ Has related a fitness education level to his or her lifestyle. ◆ Applies the concept learned correctly to an adult or sibling at home and returns the signed tasked form to the teacher.
3	◆ Completed the task form neatly. ◆ Can relate an activity to the principles of fitness. ◆ Has related a fitness education level to his or her lifestyle.
2	◆ Has completed the task sheet but has not related an activity to the principles of fitness.
1	◆ Has not completed the task sheet.
0	◆ No response or unscoreable

Note:
Teachers can have students use heart rate monitors or learn the manual way to detect heart rate. The concepts of the different levels of the Fitness Education Pyramid are important when applying the F.I.T.T. principle and can help students learn about fitness concepts and how they apply to their own bodies. The Fitness Education Pyramid at elementary, middle school or high school level can be obtained from http://www.myweb.cableone.net/lmauch/order.html

Information for Signs at Each Station:

WEIGHT MANAGEMENT ZONE—YELLOW

The bottom of the pyramid is the Weight Management Zone. This zone uses fat calories rather than carbohydrate calories for its fuel because of the time you exercise and as a result helps individuals lose weight. The workout provides a more **leisurely type** of workout and is a good workout for those concerned with weight management or with weight loss. It is effective when used as a recovery workout following an intense workout such as training for a sport. It is also good to use after an injury—it is low intensity, yet long enough, (time) to provide a beneficial workout. The Weight Management Zone is also good when **learning and perfecting new activities and skills**. This zone should be done at a frequency of six times per week, with an intensity of 40%-50% MHR, for the time of 60 minutes per day. Activities might include walking, recreational swimming, biking, volleyball, and badminton. Heart rate should be between 130-145 Beats Per Minute (BPM).

HEALTHY HEART ZONE—GREEN

The Healthy Heart Zone **strengths the heart** and gives it the opportunity to work at its optimum level with a steady, pain-free, moderate pace. This workout allows you to **accelerate the development of a specific body part by working it harder for a shorter period of time**. The intensity level, while strengthening the heart, is still at a pain-free level. The frequency of this zone is four to five times per week, at an intensity of 50%-70% MHR, for a time of 30 minutes. Activities might include moderate movement such as continuous tag games, biking, rollerblading, and team handball. Your heart rate should be between 145-170 Beats Per Minute.

THE KICK-IT ZONE—BLUE (Middle School)/THE AEROBIC ZONE (High School)

The Kick-It Zone **benefits both the heart and the respiratory system**. From this aerobic training zone, you will enhance your body's ability to **move oxygen** to, and **carbon dioxide away from, the muscle being used**. You will feel some of the discomforts of the training, but it is not painful. Your breathing will be strong, you will be working hard, and you will feel the exertion on your body. The frequency of this zone is three times per week , at an intensity of 70%-85% MHR, for a time of 15-30 minutes. Activities might include aerobics, running, working on the treadmill or ski machine, playing basketball or soccer. Your heart rate should be between 170-185 Beats Per Minute.

THE POWER ZONE—PURPLE (Middle school)/THE ANAEROBIC ZONE (High School)

The POWER ZONE allows you to **cross over and begin anaerobic training**. **Anaerobic training means without oxygen**, when there is no exchange of oxygen and carbon dioxide in your muscles. The main benefit of this training is that you increase your body's ability to **metabolize lactic acid**, allowing your muscles to train harder before crossing into the pain of lactate accumulation and oxygen debt—the pain of working out! The intensity of this training is hard. You will experience tired muscles, heavy breathing, and fatigue. This level is generally used if you are training for competition. If you are untrained or out of condition, you will feel discomfort. This zone should be at a frequency of two times per week, with an intensity of 80%-95% MHR, for a time of 5-10 minutes. Activities might include weight lifting or a series of 100-meter dashes. Your heart rate should be between 180-200 Beats Per Minute.

THE RED ZONE—RED
The RED ZONE is only for those individuals considered **extremely fit**. With this training, you cross into the anaerobic threshold and will be working in oxygen debt. The training is extremely difficult, you will feel like you cannot breathe fast enough, and that your heart is working so hard that it wants to jump out of your chest! Individuals training for **serious competition** generally use this level. Untrained or unprepared individuals who participate in these workouts will suffer great discomfort and could even suffer injury. The frequency of this zone is one time per week, with the intensity of 90%-100% MHR, and the time of one to five minutes. Activities might include jumping rope fast for one to five minutes and sprinting or running very fast for short distances. Your heart rate will be at or above 190-MHR Beats Per Minute.

The High School Fitness Education Pyramid

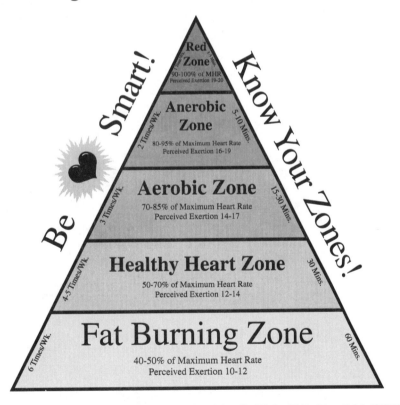

©1997, Roesler, Mauch, Schumacher, Strand, Terbizan   F.E.P. Sales & Consulting P.O. Box 201 West Fargo, N. Dak, 58078-0201

Beyond Activities

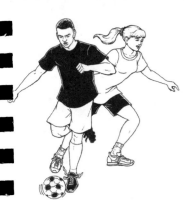

Understanding Intensity and Perceived Exertion

Cheryl Deal
2000 Southern District Middle School Teacher of the Year
Gwinnett County Public Schools—Atlanta, GA

National Standard:

Standard 4: The students will demonstrate the knowledge to monitor and adjust levels of activity to maintain or improve personal fitness level.

Students Will Learn:

1. To understand how physical activity, at varying intensity levels, influences heart rate.
2. To identify their personal perceived exertion levels during physical activity.

Teaching Strategy:

Direct instruction

How Students Will Be Organized:

◆ Assign one student to each fitness station (see station sheet).
◆ Have half of the students wear heart rate monitors (students should be familiar with using heart rate monitors).
◆ Ask the other half of the students to check their heart rates manually (six seconds and add a zero).
◆ Have students rotate after one minute at each station. Before rotating, students will record their heart rates, using Borg's scale, and their rates of perceived exertion on the back of their station sheet.
◆ Ask students, to write a descriptive phrase or sentence describing how their body feels during exertion at that station (using the key words on the back of their station sheets).
◆ Provide students who did not wear heart rate monitors in this class the opportunity to wear them during this activity the next day (all students may wear heart rate monitors if available).

Cues for Instruction:

Review Borg's scale and key words on the station sheet and what students are to record on their sheet. Instruct students to try and stay in their target heart rate zone.

Practice Activities:

Ask students to demonstrate their ability to assess their rate of perceived exertion and to hold their heart rates in their target zone, by wearing a heart rate monitor with the face of the monitor covered. Download heart rates during an activity and ask students to rate their perceived exertion on a scale of 0-10, record their responses. Have students use the information to determine if they can use their body's response to exercise to determine the intensity of that activity.

Culminating Activity:

Ask students to identify the stations at which they recorded the highest heart rates and perceived exertion rating. Discuss which stations allowed students to work in their target heart rate zone. Discuss how they would describe their bodies' physical changes at those stations.

Assessment:

Students will use heart rate data and perceived rate-of-exertion collected on their station sheets to analyze the physical changes to their bodies when they were exercising in their target heart rate zone. Students will describe how their bodies feel when they are exercising in their target zones.

*Borg Rating of Perceived Exertion (RPE) (Revised Scale)

Warm-Up/Cool Down Zone	0	Very Weak
	1	Weak
	2	A Little Weak
Target Zone	3	Moderate
	4	Strong
	5	
	6	Stronger
Working Too Hard Zone	7	Very Strong
	8	
	9	
	10	Really Strong

Key Words: **Breathing:** (deep, fast, out of breath)

Heart Rate: (fast, racing, rapid)

Fatigue: (muscles burn, feel weak, limp feeling)

Perspiration Levels: (light sweating, heavy sweating, feel hot)

*Borg, G. 1998. *Borg's Perceived Exertion and Pain Scales.* Champaign, IL: Human Kinetics

Understanding Intensity and Perceived Exertion

Fitness Stations

Stations	Heart Rate	RPE	Comments*
1. Treadmill			
2. Military Press			
3. Jump Rope*			
4. Leg Press Toe			
5. Bike			
6. Tricep Ext.			
7. Leg Lifts			
8. Bicep Curls			
9. Leg Press Toe			
10. Lateral Raise			
11. Stepper			
12. Incline Curl			
13. Chest Fly			
14. Butter Fly*			
15. Arm Ext.			
16. Bike			
17. Medicine Ball			
18. Cardio Glide			
19. Upright Row			
20. Bicep Curl			
21. Jump Rope			
22. Dips*			
23. Leg Curls			
24. Leg Ext.			
25. Bicep Curls			
26. Treadmill*			
27. Bench			
28. Cardio Glide			
29. Stepper			
30. Bench			

*Use key words from Borg's RPE chart to describe how your body feels at this station.

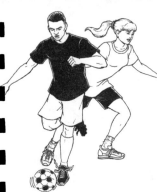

Strike and Volley

John Hichwa
1993 National Middle School Teacher of the Year
Retired—Redding Public Schools, Redding, CT

National Standards:

Standard 1: Demonstrate the skills to strike a ball over a net and against a wall, using the proper grips and stroking techniques.

Standard 2: Gain a better understanding of the skills necessary to strike a ball, keep it in play, and be able to take those new skills and practice on their own.

Standard 5: Learn to cooperate and depend on each other to learn the skills and drills.

Students Will Learn:

To strike a ball using a paddle.

Teaching Strategy:

Reciprocal

How Students Will Be Organized:

Students will work as partners with a checklist that explains how to:
- Grip the paddle.
- Volley a ball.
- Strike a bouncing ball.

The pairs will work with each other, using the paper to check their progress.

Cues For Instruction:

Listed throughout.

Practice Activities:

Each student peer checks the partner for each of the following:
- Grips
- Volleying
- Forehand and backhand stroking
- Drills for volleying and stroking

1. Grips:

- ◆ Forehand grip: Hold the paddle with the left hand and shake hands with it with the right.
- ◆ Backhand grip: Turn the forehand grip 1/4 turn counterclockwise (clockwise for left hander) until the knuckle of the pointer finger is on top.
- ◆ Continental, or volley, grip: Hold the paddle half way between the forehand and backhand grips. Practice this grip by bouncing the ball with the edge of your paddle.

Warm-up drills to practice holding the paddle correctly:

- ◆ With the forehand grip, bounce the ball on the floor at least 10 times, no higher than your waist.
- ◆ With the forehand grip, bounce the ball into the air at least 10 times, about head high.
- ◆ With the backhand grip, bounce the ball into the air at least 10 times.
- ◆ Using the continental grip, bounce the ball on the floor 10 times hitting one side of the paddle and then the other.

Check points for the grips:

- ◆ Forehand grip: Do you see a V between the index finger and thumb?
- ◆ Backhand grip: Is the knuckle of the finger on top?
- ◆ Continental grip: Can you bounce the ball on the ground with the edge of the paddle?

2. Volleying (directions for right-handed players)
Forehand volley

- ◆ Face your partner and step forward with the left foot as you throw the ball underhand to a partner. Your partner throws the ball back in like manner. Make 10 throws each.
- ◆ Throw the ball underhand at your partner's right shoulder. Your partner, facing you, catches it with his/her hand held in the position of a police officer stopping traffic. Throw and catch 10 times each.
- ◆ Throw the ball underhand to your partner's right shoulder. Your partner, in a ready position*, holds a paddle with a continental grip and volleys (punches) the ball back. Take 10 turns each.

*Ready position—Face net, knees bent, paddle held in front and cradled at throat with the other hand.

Backhand volley

- ◆ Face your partner and hold the paddle by your left shoulder and place your left hand behind the paddle. Thrower tosses the ball at the paddle. Hit the ball back as your take a step forward with your right foot. Take 10 turns each.

Check points for volleying:

- ◆ Are you facing the net in a ready position?
- ◆ Are you stepping forward with the correct foot?
- ◆ Does the punch motion begin at the shoulder?

3. Forehand and Backhand (directions for right-handed players)
Forehand

- ◆ Stand with the left side facing the net or wall, hold the right hand back at the 6 o'clock position. Drop the ball in front of your left foot, then catch the ball with your right hand while transferring your weight forward, finishing with your hand in the 12 o'clock position. Repeat 10 times.
- ◆ Hold your right hand in the 6 o'clock position as you drop the ball in front of your left foot with your left hand. Hit the ball with your right hand keeping your wrist firm. Transfer your weight forward as you strike the ball. The swing is from low (just below the waist) to high (shoulder height). Hold at the 12 o'clock position for three seconds. The partner catches the ball and strokes it back in a similar manner. Repeat 10 times.
- ◆ Hold the paddle at 6 o'clock while your partner bounces the ball to you. Gently stroke the ball back to the tosser. Take 10 turns each.

Backhand

- ◆ Stand in the ready position, holding the paddle in a backhand grip. Turn your right side to the wall as you take the paddle back to the 6 o'clock position, placing your thumb to your thigh. Step forward as you drop the ball next to your front foot, and stroke the ball toward your partner (partner catches the ball), ending in the 12 o'clock position. Switch with your partner, who strokes 10 backhands back to you.

Culminating Activity:

Volleying Drills:
Students will practice volleying using the proper grip, with each checking the other for proper hand placement. They will attempt to keep the ball in play (hitting the ball before it hits the ground), counting their consecutive hits and then attempting to better each try.

- ◆ Partners hit 10 forehand volleys to one another.
- ◆ Partners hit 10 backhand volleys to one another.
- ◆ Hit a forehand volley to your partner's backhand. Partner returns the volley to your forehand. Repeat 10 times and change positions.

Stroking Drills:
Students will practice stroking the ball against the wall, using first their forehands and then their backhands. They will attempt to hit five balls in succession, striking the ball after it hits the ground. Once that is accomplished, they will alternate forehand and backhand and attempt to hit as many as they can without error.

Game:

The partners will play a game using a net or a pair of buckets.

Partners stand on opposite sides of a net (or its substitute) and take turns putting the ball in play (to serve, players bounce the ball and hit it). A player scores a point when the other player makes an error (does not successfully return the ball back over the net after one bounce). After one player serves the ball five times, the other player will serve for five consecutive times. When one player reaches 15 points, players start a new game.

If no nets are available, both players have a bucket approximately two yards in front of them. Play begins with the serve (serve—bounce ball and hit); partners try to strike the ball on a bounce and land the ball in the other person's bucket.

Assessment:

Check points for stroking: Self-Assessment
Forehand

- ◆ Is your wrist firm as you make contact with the ball?
- ◆ Where is your paddle head at the end of the swing?
  Does it point to where you want the ball to go?
- ◆ Do you return to the ready position after each hit?

Backhand

- ◆ Does your paddle start back at the thigh when you begin the stroke?
- ◆ Are you swinging from the shoulder?
- ◆ Is your racket at the 12 o'clock position at the end of the stroke?

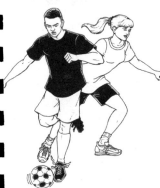

Beef Basketball

Bill Newlun
1998 National Middle School Teacher of the Year
Sisson School—Mt. Shasta, CA

National Standards:

Standard 1: Demonstrate competency in the skill of shooting a basketball.

Standard 5: Demonstrate responsible personal and social behavior
in a physical activity setting.

Students Will Learn:

The one-hand set shot by the "BEEF" method

Teaching Strategy:

Reciprocal, self-check

How Students Will Be Organized:

Students will work as partners and will have a sheet that lists and describes the BEEF shooting steps so partners can take each other through the steps using the wall, then at a basket. The partners will work with each other until they both master all four steps.

Cues For Instruction:

B—balance
E—elbows
E—eyes (aim)
F—follow through

Practice Activities:

1. Students check each other for each of the four steps from a checklist.
2. Practice at a basket with each partner shooting 3 shots while the partner watches and calls the BEEF cues as they shoot.
3. All students shooting 2-groups/per baskets. If in groups of 3's one will rebound for the shooter. The teacher reinforces the shooters; pointing out the BEEF cues they are using walking from basket to basket.
4. When shooter thinks they "got it," they call the cues off themselves and demonstrate them as they shoot.

Culminating Activity:

After this practice, the teacher introduces students to a shooting game and challenge: **The Big BEEF Challenge.**

Teachers should place seven spots in an arch pattern around each basket, the letters "BEEF" should be on four of the seven spots. When shooting from a lettered spot the shooter must say that cue (for example, "B for balance) and demonstrate it while making the shot. The rest of the shooting game is like "around the world."

Assessment:

Teachers use the "BEEF" checklist assessment as they walk behind the shooting lines to check students' use of the cues. Teachers make final assessments by comparing pre- and post-test scores on shooting skills test.

Player Info _____

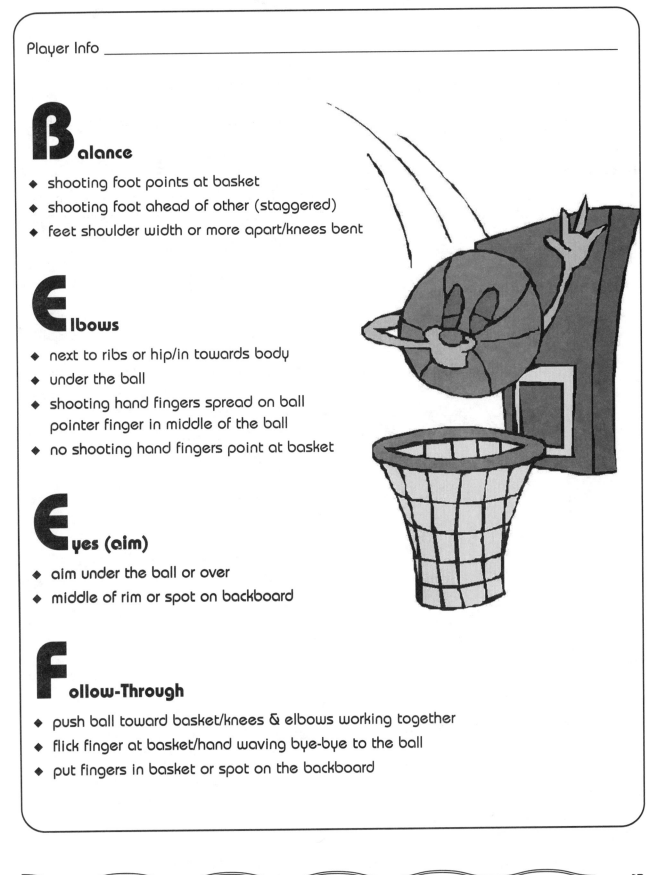

Balance

- ◆ shooting foot points at basket
- ◆ shooting foot ahead of other (staggered)
- ◆ feet shoulder width or more apart/knees bent

Elbows

- ◆ next to ribs or hip/in towards body
- ◆ under the ball
- ◆ shooting hand fingers spread on ball pointer finger in middle of the ball
- ◆ no shooting hand fingers point at basket

Eyes (aim)

- ◆ aim under the ball or over
- ◆ middle of rim or spot on backboard

Follow-Through

- ◆ push ball toward basket/knees & elbows working together
- ◆ flick finger at basket/hand waving bye-bye to the ball
- ◆ put fingers in basket or spot on the backboard

Beyond Activities

The Heart Stock Market

Shelley Paul Smith
2002 Central District Elementary School Teacher of the Year
Center for Creative Learning—Rockwood Gifted Program—Ellisville, MO

National Standards:

Standard 4: Achieve and maintain a health-enhancing level of fitness. Students will:

- Evaluate the level of exertion required to perform a variety of physical activities.
- Develop a plan to visit fitness stations in such an order as to increase personal earnings on the Heart Stock Market by applying basic fitness principles.
- Participate at fitness stations demonstrating strategies that are health enhancing and that will maintain or increase heart rate and improve personal fitness.
- Reflect on the success of their individual strategies to increase earnings on the Heart Stock Market. Analyze how varying levels of personal effort and fitness—along with the successful application of fitness principles—affect heart rate, the outcome of the activity, and ultimately personal fitness.

Standard 7: Students will understand that physical activity provides opportunity for enjoyment, challenge, self-expression, and social interaction. Students will:

- Demonstrate personal responsibility by exercising appropriately and according to the guidelines of the lesson. Demonstrate "best effort" to accomplish learning goals.
- Enjoy the challenge to think critically in an open-ended context as they exercise with peers.
- Articulate how to transfer knowledge gained from this lesson to other fitness contexts.

Students Will Learn:

To evaluate the level of exertion required to perform a variety of physical activities and develop a plan to visit fitness stations in such an order as to continuously increase their heart rate.

Teaching Strategy:

Discovery learning, integrating real-world skills, teacher acts as facilitator to help students think critically and draw conclusions.

How Students Will Be Organized:

Students will be organized at eight stations around the gym. They will choose the order in which they visit the stations.

Cues for Instruction:

Each time you raise your heart rate at a station today, you will earn "money" on the Heart Stock Market, each time your heart rate drops, you will lose money! At the end of today's lesson, you will calculate your earnings for the money you have earned. During the station exploration time, students will refer to the *Thinking Cues* task card, which will provide cues to help them make decisions about the four activities they will choose for the Heart Stock Market. Note: The teacher's task is to act as a *facilitator* to enable students to discover strategies on their own. The teacher should ask questions to elicit critical thinking from students, but refrain from *telling* them specific strategies.

Thinking Cues

- ◆ How vigorous is this activity? What are the physiological signs that show how hard your body is working?
- ◆ Where in a sequence of four would you place this activity to increase earnings on the Heart Stock Market?
- ◆ How can you use your arms to add intensity?
- ◆ Can you make your motions bigger/smaller to change your heart rate?
- ◆ How does increasing/decreasing speed affect your performance?
- ◆ How does adding weights affect intensity?
- ◆ Could you increase your body's demand for oxygen in any other ways?
- ◆ Can you identify other strategies that will increase/decrease your heart rate during this activity?

Practice Activities:

Set up eight stations around the gym that require varying amounts of aerobic effort. (Students could design the stations as part of the activity.) At least one station should require a lower level of physical effort. The first task for the students is to think about the most effective order for visiting the stations. Allow time for students to explore the stations, read task cards, and practice each activity to determine how the activity will affect heart rate. Remind students that there are many fitness principles they may incorporate to modify the heart rate. (Refer to Thinking Cues card.)

Create Task Cards for Each Station: Examples:

STATION 1 Sliding	**STATION 2** Aerobic Step	**STATION 3** Dribble & Double Jump	**STATION 4** Scooters
Slide continuously back & forth between the lines marked on the floor	Use basic step: up/up, down, down Keep pace to the music	Dribble ball 2x in place, hold the ball and jump 2x in place	Sit, kneel or lay on your stomach, move continuously around the cones
STATION 5 Partner Over/Under	**STATION 6** Line Jumping	**STATION 7** "Skip Its"	**STATION 8** Jog & Weave
One partner makes a bridge with body, other partner crawls under. Repeat continuously	Jump continuously back & forth over the line on the floor	Jump continuously over the "skip it"	Jog & Weave continuously between the cones

Culminating Activity:

◆ Students now choose the order in which they will visit stations and enter each station on the appropriate lines below the graph. Note: *There is no restriction as to how many students may visit a station at one time.* Make sure there is enough equipment if many students choose to visit the same station.

◆ Determine whether the class will palpate the pulse or use heart rate monitors. Instruct students how to plot the heart rates on the graph.

◆ Follow these steps until students have visited every station.

Set the clock. Start step music. Exercise for two minutes.

Sit down immediately in place, the teacher says: ready, count!

Enter current heart rate on the graph; connect the lines between the previous heart rate and the newest heart rate. Calculate the difference between the previous heart rate and the current one. If the heart rate increased put a (+) above the graph line. If the rate decreased place a (-) above the graph line. *(See the sample)*

For example: Resting heart rate   = 60

Current heart rate   = 90

Earnings   = +30

Move to the next station with the graph, repeat procedure.

◆ Have students calculate their earnings when all four stations have been completed. The final total is the result of adding all the increased heart rates together and subtracting any decreases in heart rate. Enter the final earnings on the line provided. (*See the sample.*) Optional: the teacher can design a "fitness-themed bank check" and the students may write themselves a "check" for their earnings on the Heart Stock Market.

Assessment:

Questioning: Reflective questioning during closure is an important assessment tool for both student and teacher. Questioning enables students to reflect on the activity, draw conclusions about the concepts involved, and transfer the day's learning to broader contexts.

◆ What factors did you consider when you decided the order in which you would visit the stations?

◆ Did your heart rate increase as you thought it might? Why or why not?

◆ What physiological signs signaled that you were working moderately or vigorously?

◆ What fitness principles did you apply to raise your heart rate at stations?

◆ We only spent two minutes at each station. How would the amount of time spent exercising affect your heart rate?

◆ Ask students to share their graphs. Is the graph a good way to assess your performance today? Explain your answer. Have the class study the differences among them. Why are they different? Did some graphs continue to show an increase in heart rate? Why? Do some show a decline in the heart rate? Why or when did the rate decrease?

◆ Analyze and share your conclusions about how a person's fitness level would affect heart rate. Would a fit person have a heart rate that goes up rapidly? Explain your answer.

◆ What would the graph of an unfit person tend to look like? Why? Today, an "unfit" person might earn more money than a "fit" person. Can you explain that?

◆ What can be learned from the Heart Stock Market that applies to lifelong fitness?

◆ Today, we participated in fitness activities, calculated heart rates, graphed heart rates, and used math to calculate earnings. We used critical thinking, logic and reasoning to make decisions. Can these skills be used in other places? Give examples and explain why the use of these skills is important in the "real" world.

Journaling: Integrate writing in physical education by asking students to respond on the back of the graph to some of the prompts in the closing questions. Assess students' ability to: meet the stated objectives, apply fitness principles, and effectively articulate what they learned and what conclusions they made after evaluating their personal plan and their performance on the Heart Stock Market.

Name _____Ima Fitkid_____   Total Earnings $ _____120.00_____

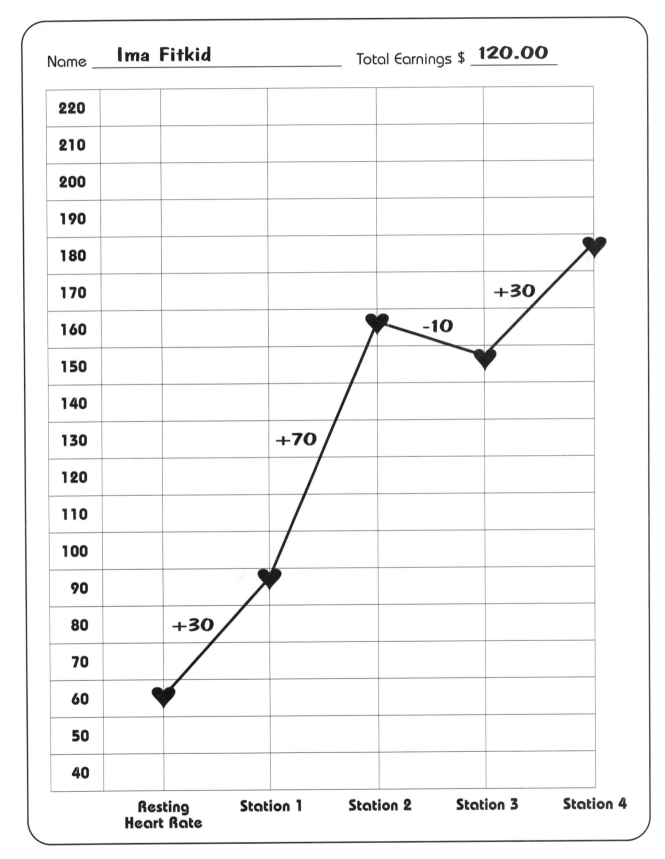

The Heart Stock Market

Name _____**Ima Fitkid**_____ Total Earnings $ ____**120.00**____

	Resting Heart Rate	Station 1	Station 2	Station 3	Station 4
220					
210					
200					
190					
180					
170					
160					
150					
140					
130					
120					
110					
100					
90					
80					
70					
60					
50					
40					

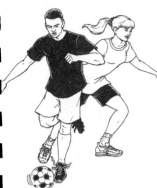

Fitness Choreography

Don Zehrung
1997 Oregon Middle School Teacher of the Year
Conestoga Middle School—Beaverton, OR
Tonia Wubbena

National Standards:

Standard 1: Require students to demonstrate a competency in a variety of locomotor and manipulative skills.

Standard 2: Apply movement concepts with emphasis on synchronization, rhythm, timing and flow.

Students Will Learn:

Student self-selected locomotor and non-manipulative skills with attention to rhythm, timing, and flow.

How Students Will Be Organized:

self-selected groups of one to five students

Teaching Strategy:

Discovery, individually designed program

Cues For Instruction:

Students will use their scoring guide (included) as their road map. References such as videos of past performances, instructional videos (hip hop steps, aerobics, Taibo), and wall charts of traditional dance steps will be provided.

Practice Activities:

The activities in this learning experience are self-directed as the students practice skills, refer to references, consult with the teacher and other students to plan the routine. Six class periods are recommended to plan and create the routine. Worksheets are provided as a guide for the groups to "script" their routines. This will enable the teacher to review the progress of each group, ask questions, and offer suggestions.

Culminating Activity:

Each group will perform their routine for the teacher. Those performances that earn an "A" may repeat the performance for the purpose of videotaping to be used as a future "reference tape."

Assessment:

Daily (formative) assessment will occur as teachers visit work groups, ask questions, and direct students to the resource center. The summative evaluation will be based upon the scoring guide.

Exercise Routine Scoring Guide

Class/Teacher _____ Grade _____

Group members:

_____ _____ _____ _____ _____

POINT TOTAL

1. Routine is 2 minutes in length _____
   4 pts. = 2 minutes or longer
   3 pts. = 1 min. 45 sec.
   2 pts. = 1 min. 30 sec.
   1 pt. = less than 1 min. 30 sec.

2. Routine is well rehearsed _____
   4 pts. = all group members synchronized, routine completely memorized
   3 pts. = most members synchronized, routine completely memorized
   2 pts. = most members synchronized, part of routine memorized
   1 pt. = some synchronization, routine not memorized

3. Routine is creative _____
   4 pts. = excellent choreography with few moves or steps repeated
   3 pts. = good choreography with several moves or steps repeated
   2 pts. = many of the moves or steps are repeated
   1 pt   = routine repeats constantly and lacks creativity

4. Routine includes 3 different movements to the side _____
   4 pts. = all 3 movements included are different and proficient
   3 pts. = the 3 movements are not different, but they are proficient
   2 pts. = 2 proficient movements that are different
   1 pt. = 1 proficient movement to the side

5. Routine includes 3 different movements forward and back _____
   4 pts. = all 3 movements included are different and proficient
   3 pts. = the 3 movements are not different, but they are proficient
   2 pts. = 2 proficient movements that are different
   1 pt. = 1 proficient movement forward and back

6. Movements go with music _____
   4 pts. = routine is in 8 count format with all movements matching music
   3 pts. = routine is in 8 count format with most movements matching music
   2 pts. = routine does not follow 8 counts, movement and music are off
   1 pt. = movement and music do not match

7. Routine includes strength activity that isolates. _____
   4 pts. = abdominals, upper arms, back, and legs
   3 pts. = 3 of the above
   2 pts. = 2 of the above
   1 pt. = 1 of the above

8. Group is smiling and making a pleasant presentation _____
   4 pts. = all group members are enthusiastic throughout the routine
   3 pts. = most members are enthusiastic throughout the routine
   2 pts. = some members are enthusiastic, some are not
   1 pt. = lack of enthusiasm shown by members of the group

9. Routine is submitted in hard copy prior to performance _____
   4 pts. = copy is comprehensive and neatly written or typed
   3 pts. = copy includes most of the choreography and is neatly written or typed
   2 pts. = copy is missing much of the routine OR is not neatly done
   1 pt. = missing information AND not legible

Total Points Possible: 36   **Your Score:** _____

33 - 36 points = A
32 points   = A-
31 points   = B+
29 - 30 points = B
28 points   = B-
27 points   = C+
25 - 26 points = C
24 points   = C-
23 points   = D+
21 - 22 points = D
20 or less   = F

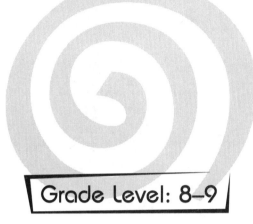

Tinikling and Jump Bands

Charlene A. Darst
2001 National Elementary School Teacher of the Year
Whitman Elementary School—Mesa, AZ

Paul W. Darst
Arizona State University—Tempe, AZ

National Standards:

Standard 1: Competency is demonstrated by the learner's ability to perform one of the three dance steps through moving poles and move the poles correctly to the music.

Standard 5: Success of the group's ability to perform the dances is dependent on each member of the group.

Students Will Learn:

Students will learn how to move the tinikling poles to the 3/4 rhythm of the music and to dance one of three variations of the tinikling step between the poles.

Teaching Strategy:

Jigsaw

How Students Will Be Organized:

Students will be organized into groups of four.
Four stations will be set up, one in each corner of the gymnasium.
One person will be sent to each corner of the gym to a specified station.
Station signs will guide the learner through the specific skill to be learned.

◆ Station number 1 is an in, in, out step.
◆ Station number 2 is a double foot in, in, out step.
◆ Station number 3 is the traditional tinikling step of in, change feet and out.
◆ Station number 4 will be the correct rhythm for the poles of out, out, slide together.

Once each individual member has learned the step at their station, they will go back to their original group and teach their sequence of steps.

Cues for Instruction:

Beginning step—Station 1

Begin with your right side to the poles. With your weight on your outside leg, hop over the pole, hop in place on the same leg, and hop back with your weight on your original leg (**over, over, back**) OR—With your right side to the pole and weight on your left foot, hop onto your right foot once over the pole, once in place and then hop back onto your left leg (**right, right, left**).

Double ins and outs—Station 2

Jump in between both poles with weight on the balls of your feet and jump again, then straddle the legs out (with one foot now on each side of the poles) for one count (**in, in, out**).

Basic tinikling step—Station 3

Right side to the poles, hop in between the poles on your right, change feet inside the poles to your left foot, hop out on the opposite side on your right foot (**in, change feet and out**)

Moving the poles—Station 4

Tap poles wide for two counts, and then slide them together for one count.

Practice Activities:

Equipment: Two wooden riders and two tinikling poles (or PVC pipe works great and is sturdier) for every group of four. If wooden riders are placed on carpet squares, it cuts down on the noise and helps to keep the riders from sliding.

Music: *We Will Rock You* for day one. Shania Twain's *Any Man of Mine* for day two, and *Shrek* #5 for the jump bands.

◆ Students will work in groups of four.
◆ All students will be practicing the beginning step over a stationary line on the floor. If lines are not available, a jump rope laid out on the floor will work fine.
◆ Step is taught and practiced without music, and then music is added. Students should lead, over a line, with both sides of the body.
◆ Basic step is taught between stationary poles.
◆ Two-foot step is taught between stationary poles.
◆ Pole rhythm is taught and practiced without dancers.
◆ While two of the group members are doing the poles, the other two group members are clapping out the rhythm.
◆ As students begin to try the step through moving poles, only one dancer should be dancing through the poles at a time. The other dancer is waiting outside the poles clapping the rhythm.
◆ Once the dancer is successful with the steps, they should take a turn moving the poles.

Add step variations:

◆ In, pivot, and out the opposite side.
◆ With one partner on each side of the poles, right hands joined, in, pivot, and out.

All of these steps can be practiced through the jump bands using a 4/4 rhythm instead of a 3/4 rhythm. Band holders wrap bands around their ankles and jump out, out, in, in.

Culminating Activity:

◆ Place tinikling poles in a tic tac toe formation by combining two sets of poles and riders. Dancers have the option of dancing through the center square, or they can move around the four poles in a clockwise or counterclockwise formation.

◆ Place poles in a horizontal side-by-side order. Dancers try to dance through the series of poles, beginning at one end of the poles and finishing at the other end.

◆ Jump band rhythm changes to 4/4 time, but by just adding a pause after they jump out the same steps can be used. With the double foot jump with the bands, it is in, in, out, out. The rhythm with the bands placed on the ankles is an out, out, together, together step.

◆ Jump bands can be placed in a vertical series. Dancers dance in one side, move out the other to the next series of jump bands, and follow the same sequence to the end. All bands must be moving in the same rhythm.

Assessment:

Students will be asked to clap the rhythm of the sticks.

Over a stationary line, students must perform one of the three required steps on command.

Their peers, using a simple peer evaluation checklist, will assess students as they work within their group.

Tinikling Peer Checklist

Name _____

Room Number _____   Teacher's Name _____

Did he/she move the poles in rhythm to the music?   ❑ YES   ❑ NO

Was he/she able to move in and out of the poles
using one of the required steps?   ❑ YES   ❑ NO

Did he/she cooperate with the group by taking turns?   ❑ YES   ❑ NO

Track & Field Fitness Routine

Charlene A. Darst
2001 National Elementary School Teacher of the Year
Whitman Elementary School—Mesa, AZ

Paul W. Darst
Arizona State University—Tempe, AZ

National Standards:

Standard 4: Students must be able to select an exercise that they can successfully perform for strengthening each component of fitness and they must also know the components of fitness. All of these concepts are necessary to maintain a health-enhancing level of physical activity.

Students Will Learn:

To make an exercise choice at each station that they can be successful, yet challenged, while performing.

Teaching Strategy:

Task signs or station signs.

How Students Will Be Organized:

Station signs will be set up in a circuit around the teaching area. Students will be divided into equal groups by sending three to four students to each station. An audio tape will be used that allows the workload to be 30 seconds at each station, with a six-second pause to move onto the next station.

Cues For Instruction:

Station signs are color coded for each fitness component. Cardiovascular endurance signs are colored red, upper body strength is coded yellow, abdominal strength signs are blue, and flexibility station signs are green. Students should be questioned as to what component of fitness they are working on.

Reinforcement should be provided for correct stretching positions and for holding the stretch for 10 counts.

As management reinforcement, students should be reinforced for jumping rope in the designated area and for jogging in the correct area and in the appropriate direction.

Reinforcement should be based on correct position and quick choices versus how many of each exercise the student completes.

Practice Activities:

Refer to attached station signs, which can be copied for personal use.

Culminating Activity:

This fitness routine in itself is a culminating activity. Students must have previous knowledge of fitness choices in order to successfully participate in this routine. This is an excellent fitness choice for the second semester of school.

Assessment:

At the conclusion of class, each squad will be asked to perform one exercise for either flexibility, abdominal strength, upper body strength or cardiovascular endurance. Teachers can ask students, "With a show of fingers, how long should you hold each stretch? What would be one flexibility exercise to get your arms ready for participating in the softball throw?

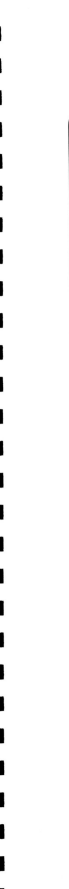

Track and Field Fitness

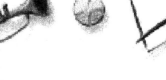

Position a cardio-vascular choice station in each corner of the teaching area. In each of these corners there should be a mat or a bench for step ups and at least 5-6 jump ropes. Establish a predetermined spot on the floor for the rope jumping and a designated jogging area. Other signs should be placed around the area as a circuit.

A music tape with intervals of 30 secs. of music followed with a 6 second pause works great for this fitness routine.

Students perform the exercise challenges while the music is playing and move to the next station on the pauses.

This routine provides students with the opportunity to choose an appropriate fitness challenge at each station.

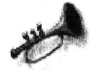

Cardiovascular Endurance

1. Jog around the outside big circle

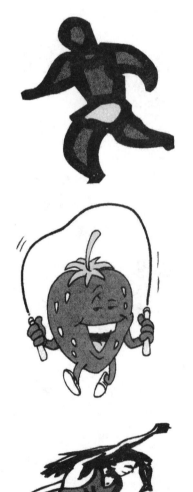

2. Jump rope inside the middle circle

3. Step up on the bench

vary your arms - punch out
punch up

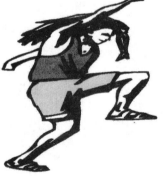

Abdominal Strength

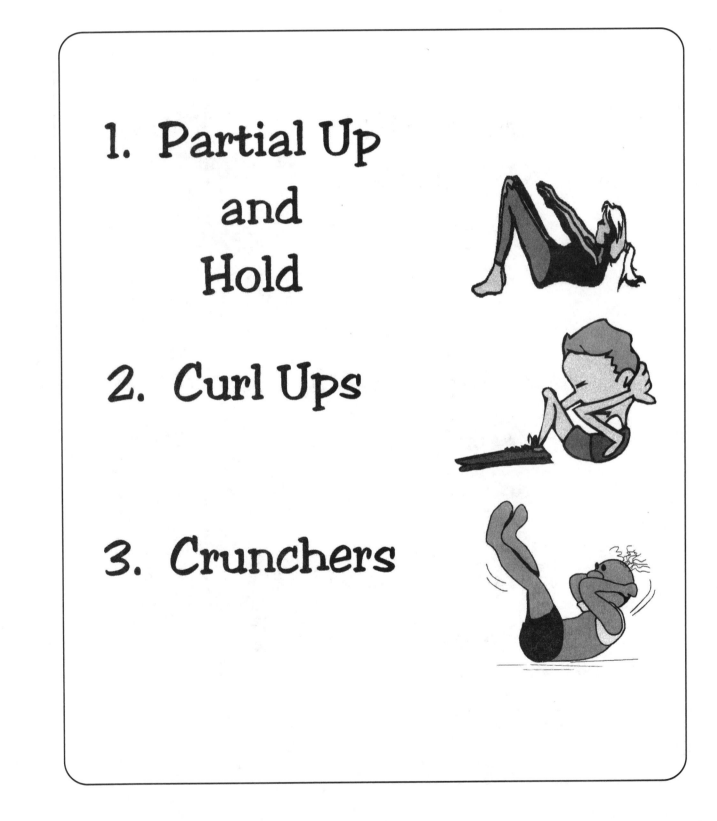

1. Partial Up and Hold

2. Curl Ups

3. Crunchers

Flexibility

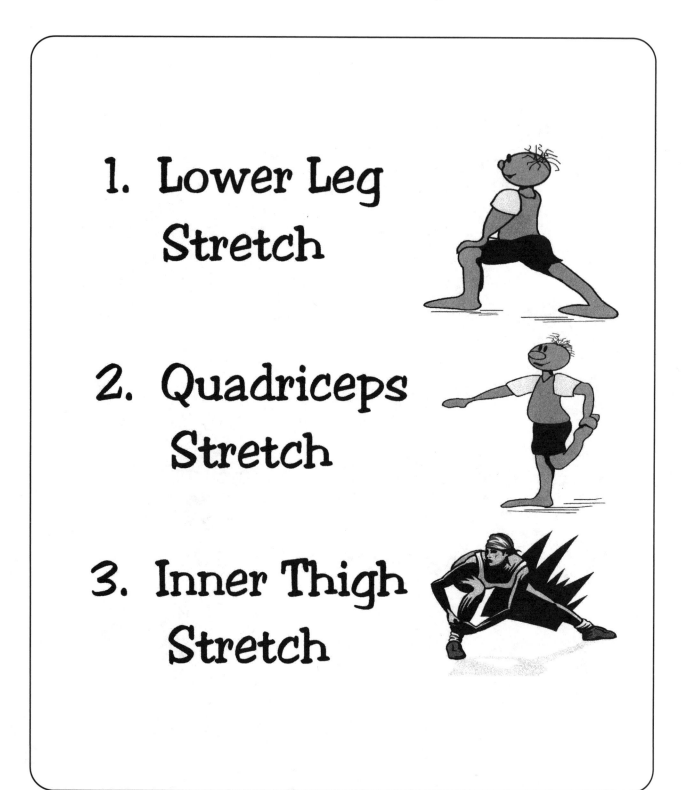

1. Lower Leg Stretch

2. Quadriceps Stretch

3. Inner Thigh Stretch

Flexibility

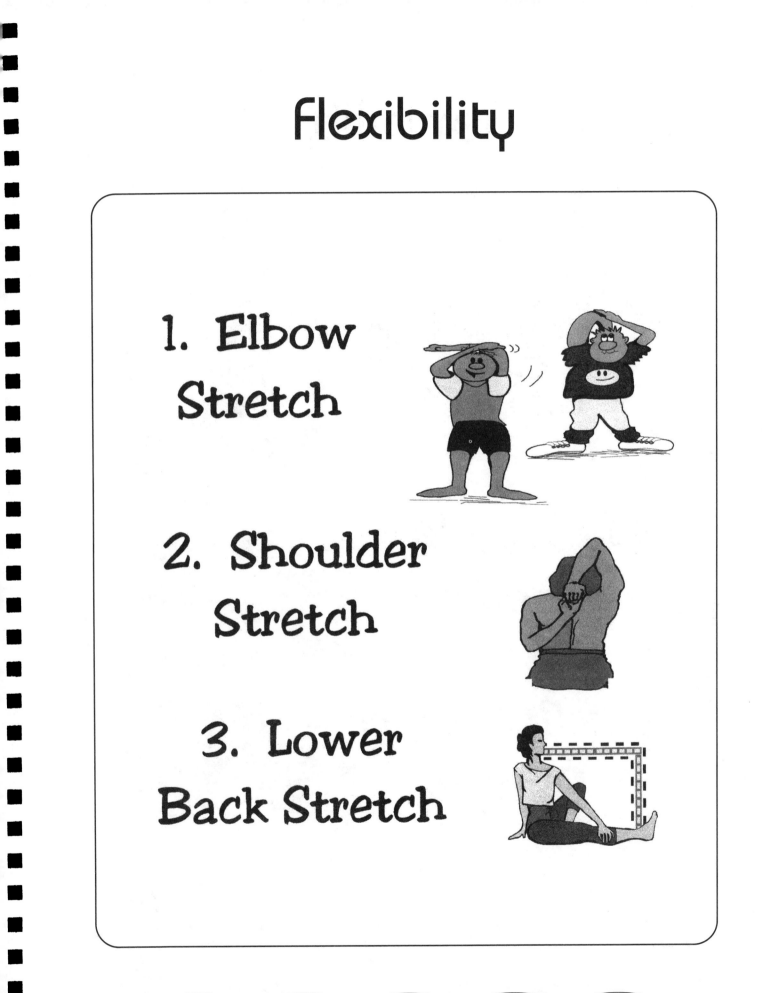

1. Elbow Stretch

2. Shoulder Stretch

3. Lower Back Stretch

Flexibility

1. Butterfly Stretch

2. Hurdle Stretch

3. Straddle Stretch

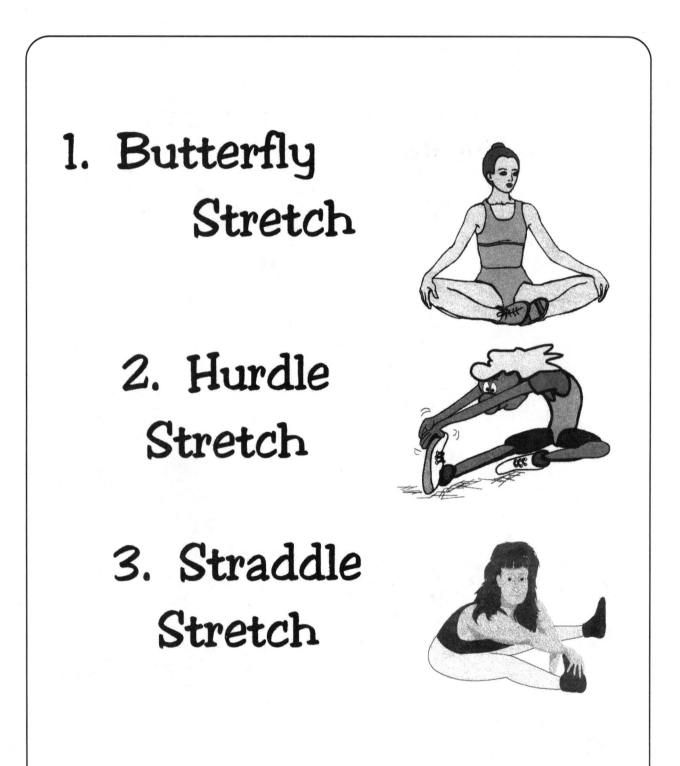

Beyond Activities

Upper Body Strength

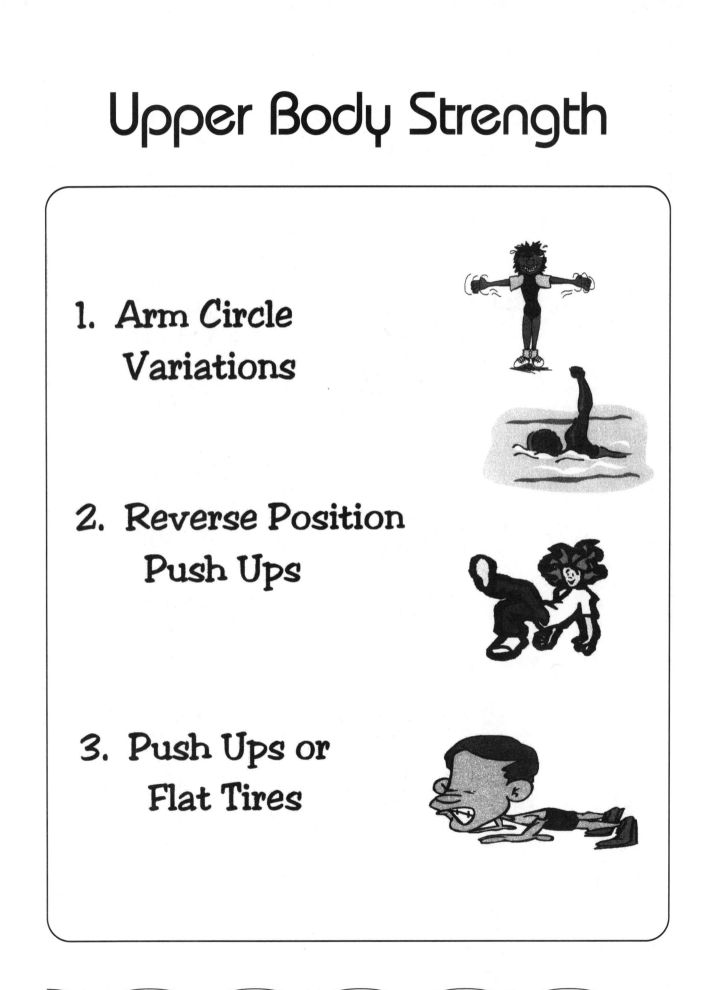

1. Arm Circle
   Variations

2. Reverse Position
   Push Ups

3. Push Ups or
   Flat Tires

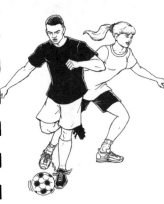

Students Creatively Leading Aerobics

Dale Kephart
2001 NASPE National Secondary School Teacher of the Year
University of Alaska Anchorage—Anchorage, AK

National Standards:

Standard 1: Students learn specific aerobic steps and perform a routine and students are assessed on the proficiency of the routine. Students should show competency in the creative portion of the assignment.

Standard 4: The students remain active for 30+ minutes and incorporate the following components of fitness: cardiorespiratory, body composition, and flexibility.

Standard 5: The students take on a leadership role, cooperate with others, and show honest, on-task behavior following the assignment and working in group settings.

Students Will Learn:

◆ How to create and teach an aerobic routine—which has fun movements performed to motivating music—to peers.
◆ How to develop social skills by interacting in small groups.
◆ How to create movements beyond the basic steps learned.

Teaching Strategy:

◆ Direct, command style for the lesson directions.
◆ Jigsaw teaching of aerobic routine.
◆ Cooperative, student-lead activities during activity.

Cues for Instruction:

◆ Teach leaders routine parts in small groups. Count out steps with word cues. Give students paper with routine and cue words written on it to take back to their groups.
◆ Verbal, positive cues as to students' leadership within their groups.
◆ Recognize groups working hard and on-task.

How Students Will Be Organized:

Once the students have learned the basics of aerobic movements, they can create on their own. Students need a basic background of a variety of aerobic movements before they assume leadership and develop new ideas. Teachers can start by letting students create short segments of movement in a variety of situations and then let them explore teaching each other and becoming creative with longer aerobic routine assignments.

Practice Activities:

This lesson assumes that the students already know the basic aerobic steps used in the lesson.

Locomotor Patterns—Aerobic Routine: Locomotion: Student-Centered Teaching in Cooperative Groups

◆ Teachers can set up a teaching area for students to come to learn the routine parts.

◆ Teachers can divide the class into groups of four: Count off each person— 1,2,3,4.

◆ Class: Warm up walking around the gym. Call leader #1 to the teaching area to learn Part I of the aerobic routine.

◆ Each group finds a place to work in the gym. Leader #1 teaches their group Part I of the routine.

◆ Leader #2 goes to the teaching area and learns part II of the routine while Leader #1 does stretches with the group.

◆ Leader #2 teaches their group Part II of the routine.

◆ Leader #3 goes to the teaching area and learns part III of the routine while Leader #2 has the group practice Part I & II together.

◆ Leader #3 teaches the group Part III of the routine.

◆ Leader #4 goes to the teaching area and learns part IV of the routine while Leader #3 has the group practice Part I, II and III together.

◆ Leader #4 teaches the group Part IV of the routine.

◆ Leader #4 has the group practice the whole routine, repeating it four times.

◆ Each leader #1-4 takes turns leading the group through the routine.

When the leaders learn the routine, they should receive their part in written form to take back to their groups in case they need to refer to it. The directions for the group are included.

Routine—Part I (32 counts):	Verbal Cues:

Leader #1:

- Walk forward R, L, R, L (roll arms)   "Do the locomotion"
- March R, L, R, L in circle to R   "Reach for the stars"
  (arms reach upward 4 times)
- Walk backward R, L, R, L (roll arms)   "Do the locomotion"
- March R, L, R, L in circle to L   "Reach for the stars"
  (arms reach upward 4 times)
- Side shuffle step to R (roll arms & step side R,   "Do the locomotion"
  close L, step side R, close L)
- March R, L, R, touch L in circle to R   "Reach for the stars"
  (arms reach upward 4 times)
- Side shuffle step to L (roll arms & step side L,   "Do the locomotion"
  close R, step side L, close R)
- March L, R, L, touch R in circle to L   "Reach for the stars"

Lead warm-up stretches when leader #2 goes to learn Part II.

Routine—Part II (32 counts):	Verbal Cues:

Leader #2:

- Skip forward: Step R forward and hop, step L   "Locomotion skips"
  forward & hop (arms swing in opposition)
- Jump crossing R in front of L (arms cross   "Locomotion jump jacks"
  in front of body, low, fists closed). Jump
  legs out to side (arms horizontal to sides,
  fists closed). Jump feet together, then
  clap two times quickly.
- Skip backward: Step R backward & hop, step   "Locomotion skips"
  L backward and hop (arms swing in opposition)
- Do jump section described above.   "Locomotion jump jacks"
- Slide to the R four times (roll arms)   "Locomotion slides"
- Do jump section described above.   "Locomotion jump jacks"
- Slide to the L four times (roll arms)   "Locomotion slides"
- Do jump section described above.   "Locomotion jump jacks"

Lead Parts I & II together when leader #3 goes to learn Part III.

Students Creatively Leading Aerobics

Routine—Part III (32 counts):
Leader #3:

	Verbal Cues:

◆ Cross step forward R, ball change (transfer weight to L foot and back to R while snapping fingers to R side of body).

"Groovy locomotion"

◆ Cross step forward L, ball change (transfer weight to R foot and back to L while snapping fingers to L side of body).

◆ Repeat cross step on R as described above.

◆ Repeat cross step on L as described above.

◆ Three-step turn to R, touch L (step R to R side, half-turn R and step L, half-turn R and step R, touch L foot beside R) and clap.
Three-step turn to L, touch R (step L to L side, half-turn L and step R, half-turn L and step L, touch R foot beside L) & clap.

"Turning locomotion"

◆ Repeat the whole sequence.

"Groovy locomotion"
"Turning locomotion"

Do Parts I, II & III together when leader #4 goes to learn Part IV.

Routine—Part IV (32 counts)
Leader #4:

Verbal Cues:

◆ Two-step to the R (step forward R, bring L foot behind R and step forward R (roll arms and flip up R arm at a right angle—flip head R)

"Shuffle locomotion"

◆ Two-step to the L (step forward L, bring R foot behind L and step forward L (roll arms and flip up L arm at a right angle -flip head L)

◆ Repeat two-step six more times to R, L, R, L, R, L.

◆ During these eight two-steps, form a line and have leader #1 lead the line around the gym. Be safe and "snake around" other groups.

◆ On two-step # 7 and 8, organize the line back into original formation to begin routine again.

Do Parts I, II, III & IV together as a complete routine. Then repeat the whole routine several times until the music stops.

Group Practice

Teacher stops group practice. Restart the music and culminate the lesson with all groups performing their routine at the same time.

Cool-down stretches within groups. Leader #1 leads the exercises.

Routine Testing For Proficiency:

Each group will perform their aerobic routine for a teacher assessment at the next class session. There will be a five-minute practice period. The evaluation will be based upon:

◆ Execution of routine
  o Steps performed correctly
  o Arm movements performed correctly
◆ Rhythm
  o Routine performed in rhythm to the music
  o Correct counts for each routine part
◆ Positive attitude
  o Enjoy doing the routine
  o Move with positive energy

Culminating Activity:

Creative Assignment For The Whole Group: Send a leader to get equipment for each person in the group. Design movements with the equipment while doing the aerobic routine. Each group will have different equipment. The steps must stay the same, but the equipment will determine what the arms and body do.

Equipment: Four of each different type of equipment. Ideas include: Grip dot balls, volley special superskin soccer ball, jump ropes, foam football, juggling scarves or objects, tambourines, hula hoops, dancing colors scarves, dancing rainbow hoops, rainbow ribbon wands, lummi sticks, basketballs. Use your imagination with equipment.

Create quickly and practice!!

Assessment:

Show Time: With groups spread out (form a square in the gym facing into center), have each group "show off" their routine doing a round robin around the gym—one group at a time so we can appreciate everyone's routine and creativity. The teacher will do a quick assessment to check for the following:

◆ Creativity
  o Using the equipment in a specific pattern while doing the routine (as evidenced by the group looking the same with the equipment patterns)
  o Fun ideas with the equipment

Name				
Execution (20)				
Rhythm (10)				
Positive Attitude (10)				
Creativity (10)				
TOTAL POINTS: (40)				

A = 40 - 36 points   D = 27 - 24 points
B = 35 - 32 points   F = 23 & below
C = 31 - 28 points

Use the following numbers to score the groups:
    Always: Place a 3 in the column
    Most of the time: Place a 2 in the column
    Sometimes: Place a 1 in the column

Group #	1	2	3	4	5	6	Comments
On task—moving quickly							
Cooperating with everyone							
Leadership by everyone							
Honest and responsible							
TOTAL							

A = 12 - 11 points
B = 10 - 9 points
C = 8 - 6 points
D = 5 - 4 points

Beyond Activities

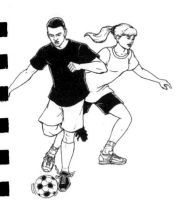

Discovering Agility in Soccer

Elaine Lindsay
1996 National High School Teacher of the Year
Retired/Baltimore County Public Schools

National Standards:

Standard 2: Applies movement concepts and principles to the learning and development of motor skills.

Students Will Learn:

To identify the skill related fitness component of agility as it is displayed in a soccer game and evaluate their own agility level, and the agility levels of classmates.

Teaching Strategy:

Peer teaching

How Students Will Be Organized:

The students will be divided into groups of approximately four to six students.

Cues For Instruction:

Describe and demonstrate the components of agility:

- Starting position: A stationary position before the take-off or a movement as preparation for take off.
- Take-off: The movement involved when leaving the starting position.
- Moving in space: Flight in the air or moving on the ground from point A to point B.
- End position: Landing after a flight to the rest position at the end of movement on the ground.
- Touch and go: When agility tasks are continuous, the end position serves as the starting position for continuous movement and the performance of a sequence of movements.

Practice Activities:

◆ Review the definition of agility (ability to change direction quickly).

◆ Discuss the heredity connection of skill-related fitness.

◆ Assign a body part to each group (sole of foot, instep, heel of foot, knee, head, chest).

◆ Instruct each group to develop a soccer drill that would have the students work on the agility of that body part.

◆ Have each group teach the drill to the rest of the class and allow the groups to practice the drill.

Culminating Activity:

Following participation in agility drills, students will participate in small (four players per team) soccer games, rotating teams as time allows. Focus of the games will be on identifying which skills require agility.

Assessment:

Students will list the soccer skills that used agility during the soccer games. Students will appraise each team member's level of agility and give examples of the skills that were performed by that team member. See attached form.

Agility Evaluation

Team Members: List the names of your team members, putting your name in block 1.

Soccer Skills that Utilized Agility	1	2	3	4	5
Passing					
Dribbling					
Receiving					
Tackling					
Dodging					
Heading					
Trapping with foot					
Trapping with leg					
Trapping with chest					
Other					

Criteria for Evaluation of Agility:

3 = Demonstrated above average agility when performing this skill

2 = Demonstrated average agility when performing this skill

1 = Agility level hampered the performance of this skill

0 = No opportunity to observe

Beyond Activities

Jump Rope School

Carol Martini
2002 National High School Teacher of the Year
Andover High School—Andover, MA

National Standards:

Standard 5: Demonstrate responsible personal and social behavior in physical activity settings. Students will:

- ◆ Provide encouragement and support to allow "concerned" individuals to give their best efforts.
- ◆ Take responsibility to act as a leader if the group needs it.
- ◆ Learn that part of a group problem solving process involves listening.
- ◆ Have the opportunity to understand and accept feelings of both "success" and "failure" as part of the group.
- ◆ Cheer outstanding accomplishments of teammates.
- ◆ Be able to identify positives (as well as negatives) with regard to peer influence.

Standard 6: Understands and respects differences among people in physical activity settings. Students will:

- ◆ Learn that a variety of ages, skill levels, body types, and both genders can work together to achieve success with this activity.
- ◆ Select, successfully and compassionately, the individual to swing the rope with the instructor.
- ◆ Begin to recognize the role that this physical activity plays in getting to know and understand others.
- ◆ Have the opportunity to demonstrate, verbally and nonverbally, cooperation with all peers.
- ◆ Have the opportunity to develop strategies to include "reluctant" participants.
- ◆ Practice being considerate of the differences of others.

Standard 7: Experience the enjoyment, challenge, self-expression, and social interaction of physical activity. Students will:

- ◆ Experience a new, exciting and interesting class challenge, with each grade level.
- ◆ Feel a tremendous sense of accomplishment when a grade level is successfully mastered.

- Value this activity as a great bonding experience for a group.
- Learn that in this activity, the girls in class are often the skill experts, which gives them the opportunity to take the lead in successfully coaching teammates.
- Have the opportunity to contribute meaningfully to the achievement of the team.

Students Will Learn:

To enhance their communication, cooperation, and problem-solving skills. Students' confidence, trust, communication, and leadership skills will be put to the test as well as their ability to value the successful skills it takes to work together as a group.

Teaching Strategy:

Guided discovery

How Students Will Be Organized:

The entire class is lined up single file (double file if the class is exceptionally large) on one side of a 32' nylon jump rope. The instructor holds one end, a student "swinger" holds the other end. The swinger changes with each grade level achieved.

Cues For Instruction:

Teachers ask:

- How will you decide who will go first?
- How will you decide who will go last?
- What is the biggest difficulty that your team is facing with this challenge?
- Is there any way you can make the problem more manageable?
- How did the team react to a student who made a mistake?
- What kind of feedback could (would, should) be given to:
    1. make teammates feel valued?
    2. keep struggling teammates invested in the challenge?
    3. help teammates who need it?

Practice Activities:

Teachers explain that:

◆ The class will have the opportunity to "graduate" from high school (perhaps even college) according to their ability—as a class—to achieve jump rope school success.

◆ Some grade levels will allow each person to move onto the next grade based strictly on individual ability to perform the challenge (in reality, this is a practice opportunity for students to "prove" that they are competent, and to relieve any self-imposed pressure). These grades are written in blue below.

◆ Other grade levels will only allow students to move on as an entire class (all or none). These grades are written in red below.

◆ As the rope swings toward the class, the students must pass through the rope as follows:

Elementary School

K - each student runs, one at a time, through the middle (unlimited swings between students)

1 - each person runs under the rope, one swing per customer

Double Promotion

3 - with partner (unlimited swings)

4 - one swing per pair

Middle School

6 - in and make 1 jump (unlimited swings)

7 - in and make 1 jump, one swing per customer

Double Promotion

High School

9 - with partner, make 1 jump and out (unlimited swings)

10 - with partner, 1 jump (one swing per pair)

11 - individually make 2 jumps (unlimited swings)

12 - with partner make 2 jumps (one swing per pair)

Master's Degree

Entire class together—make a minimum of 3-5 jumps

Ph.D.

Alternating jumpers

Culminating Activity:

Any grade from high school to college can be used as a culminating activity for the class. Ideally the skills students demonstrate in this lesson will serve as a foundation for future group problem-solving activities.

Assessment:

Student learning can be assessed in a number of ways depending on instructor preference—such as:

◆ teacher observation of the group dynamics and interactions of students
◆ students' debriefing responses
◆ student reflection paper

Teachers can highlight positive techniques, methods, strategies, character qualities, etc. on a wall for future class reference.

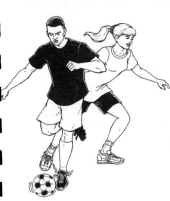

Cooperative Beating Hearts

Karen M. Roesler
1998 National Secondary School Teacher of the Year
Fargo South High School—Fargo, ND

National Standards:

Standard 4: Set HR zones on an individual basis, taking into account personal fitness
levels of each student.

Standard 5: Learn to take responsibility, within a group, for successful completion
of the classroom tasks.

Students Will Learn:

To analyze personal activity levels during various activities.

Teaching Strategy:

Cooperative groups with assigned responsibilities

How Students Will Be Organized:

Students will be in cooperative groups of four. Each group member is numbered
from one to four. Each member of a group will have a specific responsibility for
that group:
1 – Equipment manager
2 – Data manager
3 – Technology aid
4 – Data scorekeeper

Cues for Instruction:

Heart rate (HR) monitor operation, comments specific to each team member's
responsibility for the day

Practice Activities:

◆ Utilize HRM for various activities prior to unit for ease of operation
◆ Recalling HRM data
◆ Charting HRM data in Personal Portfolio

Culminating Activity:

All teammates will wear assigned HR Monitor, or for large classes half the students can wear HR monitors on Monday and Wednesday; the other half can wear them on Tuesday and Thursday. Each day the students will gather different HR data for their cooperative group score.

Day 1: Average HR of teammates

Day 2: Time in HR Zone added to time above zone

Day 3: Discard the lowest average HR for team, add remaining three and calculate the average

Day 4: Time in zone plus time above zone minus time below zone

Activities for this unit may vary: An example would be 4 x 4 Ultimate disk, soccer, or other similar 4 x 4 games.

Assessment:

Cooperative teams will set an HR monitor goal for that day's specific activity. Team goal will be placed on data sheet prior to the start of activity. Scorekeepers will meet after daily data has been recorded and assign the team a score based on group goal set and actual HR data collected.

Cooperative Team Assessment

Each student may complete a Self-Assessment or Cooperative Team Assessment

Date	Activity	Team/Individual Heart Rate Goal	Heart Rate Data	Comments

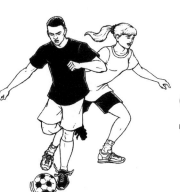

Scramble Fitness Dice

Dale Kephart
2001 National Secondary School Teacher of the Year
University of Alaska Anchorage—Anchorage, AL

National Standards:

Standard 4: The students remain active for 30+ minutes and incorporate the following components of fitness: cardiorespiratory, muscular strength and endurance, body composition, and flexibility.

Standard 5: The students take on a leadership role, cooperate with other students, and show honest, on-task behavior following the activity lists and working in the group settings.

Students Will Learn:

1. To practice fitness activities already learned.
2. To develop leadership and cooperation within a small group.
3. To show responsible personal and social behaviors.

Teaching Strategy:

- ◆ Direct, command style for the lesson directions.
- ◆ Cooperative, student-lead activities during activity.

Cues for Instruction:

- ◆ Verbal, positive cues as to students' behavior within their group relating to their leadership, cooperation, and responsibility levels.
- ◆ Recognize groups working hard at their fitness activities for motivation to be honest and on-task.

How Students Will Be Organized:

The teacher will:

- ◆ Prepare signs and set up for the following activities:

    Shuttle pass with the CatchBall & 2 cones. (CatchBall is a catching device with spokes that are numbered on the ends. Frisbees could also be used and divided into sections with numbers written on them)

    Push Ball & 2 cones (or any light, large ball or float-r-balls that can be kept up in the air easily)

- Place the following equipment in center of gym for access by students:
  - Jump ropes
  - Mats for exercises scattered in various places for activities
  - Mats folded to add height for triceps dips
  - Hula hoops
  - Balls for dribbling
- Organize class into six groups and explain activity.
- Give each group one "Scramble" paper and colored marker. The paper has a list of fitness activities that the groups will follow. There are six different papers for each class, each group's activities are the same, but starts with a different exercise. Teachers should leave about three activities between each groups starting exercise, so they will start with different equipment. (Using different colored paper for each group is a good idea.)

Practice Activities:

The students are to follow the exercises and activities *in order*. All activities have been performed in class previously. The equipment is spread out throughout the gym. Each group is to get the equipment as needed, or go to an area marked for a specific activity. They must move as a group.

- Group moves at its own pace!
- Students are to be responsible and watch for other students and groups.
- Students should return the equipment back to its area when finished.
- Groups come to the marked area in the center of the gym, after each exercise or activity, roll the foam dice (or use regular dice on a table) and a designated honest, responsible leader in each group writes the dice # in the blank on the paper. (The teacher or a student unable to participate can also fulfill the roll of writing in the numbers). Teachers should be available to guide the groups with leadership, cooperation, and on-task behavior while moving around the gym.

Culminating Activity:

- ◆ When groups are finished or at the end of class they add up their points and write the total at end of paper. If total is wrong, penalty is 10 pts. If the group does not stay together the penalty is five points.
- ◆ Winner: Highest total = "Luck of the Dice" Teachers can check papers and announce winner at the end of class or next class session.
- ◆ Hints for students:
  - Stay on task and move quickly. If you waste time, you won't get as many exercises done.
  - Cooperate and allow all members of the group to roll the dice.
  - Let everyone in the group lead. A different student should read the exercises and lead the group as you move through the list.
  - Be honest. Do the correct exercises and numbers as a group.
  - Check your math to make sure the total is correct

Following is a copy of the activity paper and group assessment students can use to score.

Scramble Fitness—Workout, Roll the Dice, and Look for the Lucky Winner

Each **team (all individuals)** must do the exercises **(in order)**. Go to the area where the equipment is to perform the activity. If no equipment is needed, find a clear space for your group to work. After each exercise, report to the marked dice area. Roll the dice **once** for a score and write your score in the blank space provided.

_____ Jog one lap around the outside of the gym.

_____ Perform 15 curl ups with bent knees.

_____ Put hula hoop on floor. Group gets in a push up position with hands on outside of hoop. Walk both hands inside the hoop, then back out 20 times.

_____ Jump with a single jump rope 50 times.

_____ Form a circle, join hands, skip in a circle & sing "Mary Had a Little Lamb" or "Ring Around the Rosy."

_____ Perform 30 crossover (oblique) wall curl ups (15 to R, 15 to L). Knees are bent, feet up on wall.

_____ Perform two sets of 5-10 push ups regular or on knees (your level).

_____ Pass the CatchBall in a shuttle formation. Divide group in two and line up at the two cones facing each other. Throw the CatchBall to the individual at the other cone and run to the end of the opposite line. Each time you catch, yell out the number you caught it on, add it to the team total and say total = _____. Continue until your team score = 100.

_____ Grab a jump rope for each person, the group skips rope one lap around the outside of the gym.

_____ Form a circle and hook feet. Perform curl up while singing "Row, Row, Row Your Boat" three times. Get louder each time.

_____ Perform 10 triceps dips, (crab position with hands on a folded mat—bend elbows and straighten).

_____ Hold one jump rope—everyone should have a hand on it—and jog one lap around the outside of the gym.

_____ Perform five clap push ups (your level of push up position).

_____ Run in place with hands in front of body, lift knees high enough to touch hands. Say the alphabet out loud from A to Z.

_____ Shuffle step to the side one lap around the outside of the gym. Change sides halfway around.

_____ Cooperate to keep the PushBall (or any light, large ball) up in the air while moving between the two cones two times, finishing at the cone you started at. If you drop the ball, start over.

_____ Perform an isometric wall sit for 20 seconds. Count one thousand 1, etc. out loud.

_____ Form a circle. Perform 20 jumping jacks and count out loud.

_____ Dribble a ball one lap around the outside of the gym.

_____ Hold a hula hoop in the middle of the group-everyone helps. Counting out loud, slide clockwise 10 times, then counterclockwise 10 times.

_____ **TOTAL SCORE**

Evaluate Your Group's Performance Today!

Evaluate your group's performance today during the activity:

Use the following numbers to score your group:

Always:	Place a 3 in the Always column
Most of the time:	Place a 2 in the Most of the Time column
Sometimes:	Place a 1 in the Sometimes column

Our group was:	Always	Most of the time	Sometimes	Total
On task—moving quickly				
Cooperating with everyone				
Lead by everyone				
Honest and responsible				

Add totals up and place in blank: Score Total = _____

Names in Group:

1. _____   4. _____
2. _____   5. _____
3. _____   6. _____

Assessment:

Students assess their groups at the end of the class activity. See table above on the student's activity sheet.

Teachers can keep a record of observation to compare with the group evaluations:

Use the following numbers to score the groups:

Always:	Place a 3 in the column
Most of the time:	Place a 2 in the column
Sometimes:	Place a 1 in the column

Group #	1	2	3	4	5	6	Comments
On task—moving quickly							
Cooperating with everyone							
Lead by everyone							
Honest and responsible							
TOTAL							

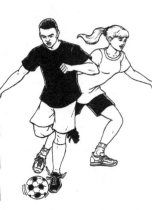

Changing Intensity Levels to Fit Your Fitness Program

Elaine Lindsay
1996 National High School Teacher of the Year
Retired/Baltimore County Public Schools

National Standards:

Standard 4: Learn the information to achieve and maintain a health enhancing level of physical fitness.

Students Will Learn:

1. To identify ways to modify exercises in order to apply the principle of overload.
2. To evaluate their personal levels of fitness.
3. To design a personal exercise program utilizing intensity level differences presented by their peers.

Teaching Strategy:

Critical thinking and group sharing

How Students Will Be Organized:

The students will be divided into groups of four to six students. After each group presents three levels of an exercise, the students will work individually to construct an exercise program that will be personally beneficial.

Cues For Instruction:

◆ Review the definition of overload and the ways that overload can be achieved (changing the FITT). This lesson will focus on changing levels of intensity. Each student is to determine the intensity level of each exercise that will promote fitness improvement via the Principle of Overload.

◆ The students are aware of the terms "set" and "reps," as they apply to an exercise session.

Practice Activities:

- ◆ Assign an exercise to each group, such as curl-ups, push-ups, hamstring stretch, leg exchange, wall sit, or jump rope.
- ◆ Instruct each group to develop three levels of the exercise. Level 1 should be able to be performed by all students in the class. Level 2 should be able to be performed by most of the people in the class. Level 3 should be able to be performed by only a few students in the class.
- ◆ Have each group demonstrate the three levels to the rest of the class. Students should practice the three levels, determining which intensity level is appropriate to apply the principle of overload to their fitness program.

Culminating Activity:

Students perform repetitions and several sets of each of the demonstrated exercises. Utilize music as a motivational accent.

Assessment:

Students will submit a list of the exercises, level, sets, and reps in an order that they will be able to perform. Following performance of the series of exercises, students will evaluate the program as to its ability to maintain or improve their fitness levels.

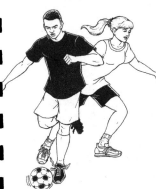

Score on Skill

Kathleen A. Thornton
1996 National Middle School Teacher of the Year
Belair High School—BelAir, MD

National Standards:

Standard 2: Apply the concept of passing while practicing the forearm pass.

Standard 5: Exhibit appropriate social behavior as students work with others to achieve the objectives of the forearm pass.

Students Will Learn:

To execute a forearm pass to a stationary or moving target.

Teaching Strategy:

Reciprocal

How Students Will Be Organized:

The students will begin in partners and then will be organized into groups of three.

Cues For Instruction:

- ◆ Feet shoulder width apart,
- ◆ Weight forward on the balls of the feet,
- ◆ Bend knees,
- ◆ Eyes on the ball,
- ◆ Receive on left side of the body,
- ◆ Straight and simple,
- ◆ Platform slanted toward target.

Practice Activities:

- ◆ Partner reciprocal practice: Player one tosses the ball to player two, who executes a forearm pass back to player one, who should not have to take more than one step in any direction. The catcher calls one cue for each forearm pass attempt. The goal is for the passer to complete 20 out of 25 passes while the cue coaching occurs. After 25 passes, players switch jobs.
- ◆ Partners pass to each other to accumulate 50 passes. Each partner calls out one of the cues as they practice. This way players are constantly reminded of the instructional cues needed to be successful.

- In groups of three, one person tosses a ball over the net to the receiver who performs a forearm pass to a third person positioned at the net. This third person is the coach, who gives correctional feedback and also catches the ball. Partner checking is essential. After all three partners have been successful they rotate again with a serve rather than a toss.
- In the group of three, one person serves to the other two who practice calling the ball and then with a forearm pass must try to get it into one of three cans or buckets, which are located in front of the net. Two points can be awarded for each ball in the can...this can be a great "cut-throat" activity where the server serves 10 and the two receivers try to accumulate as many points as possible. Each person gets to serve 10 and each remaining pair gets a chance to accumulate points.

Culminating Activity: Score On Skill

This activity is a three-on-three game. The goal of the activity is to use the forearm pass to receive the serve and put it into playing position for a teammate. The serving team earns three points each time they are able to complete the sequence, which includes a good serve and a forearm pass to the middle front position. More points are earned for completing the play: one point for a two-touch play, 2 points for a three-touch play. No points are earned if the ball is not passed to the setter. One additional point is awarded to the team who wins the rally. Serves alternate.

Assessment:

The students assess partners during the practice activities. The teacher uses the checklist sheet to assess the students as they work on the culminating activity.

Teacher Checklist Forearm Pass

Each individual will be given three trials to properly perform a forearm pass and hit the target. Teacher will review with students the proper cues before the trials begin.

Name	Stance Knees/Arms	Execution Straight/Simple	Ball to Target	Follow Through

Score on Skill

Beyond Activities

Archery Made Simple, and Maybe Golf?

Susan P. Kogut
1985 National Secondary School Teacher of the Year
Retired K-12 Physical Educator

National Standards:

Standard 1: The students will demonstrate competency in the skill of shooting an arrow.

Standard 5: The success of one student is dependent on another

Students Will Learn:

The seven shooting steps of archery
To shoot an arrow

Teaching Strategy:

Reciprocal

How Students Will Be Organized:

Students will be in partners and will have a sheet with the 7 shooting steps listed and described so that they can take each other through the steps using a large stretch band to draw and release. The students will work with each other until each has all 7 steps.

Cues For Instruction:

- ◆ Stand square
- ◆ Elbow up
- ◆ Squeeze shoulder blades together
- ◆ Open fingers
- ◆ Freeze

More specific cues are listed on the partner assessment sheet.

Practice Activities:

- ◆ Each student "peer checks" their partner for each of the 7 shooting steps
- ◆ Students practice at targets with each partner shooting 3 arrows while the other partner watches from a safe distance behind. The non-shooting partner

calls the 7 shooting steps, and the shooting partner calls the cues while shooting. Partners retrieve arrows and reverse.

- ◆ All students shoot 6 arrows on their own. The teacher walks back and forth in the back of the shooters reinforcing the 7 shooting steps and cues.
- ◆ All students shoot 6 arrows and call off the steps and cues to themselves trying for the center of the target and self analyzing each shot.
- ◆ All students shoot 6 arrows each and begin to add up a score based on the value of each of the color rings.

Culminating Activity:

After the teacher assigns a point value for each of the circles, the 4 students at each target shoot rounds of 6 per person and add the scores together as a group. The scores can be compared per target.

As the teams finish the team totals, they can trade in the target face for another challenge. An example of this would be a tic-tac-toe (on tagboard). One team of 4 would be the X and another would be the O. After a round of shooting, the arrows are removed and replaced by the little x's and o's, supplied by the teacher.

After the various target faces have been used, the shooting line can be moved back so that the distance is greater. The students can go through the same process at the new distance.

Assessment:

The "peer" assessment along with the teacher assessment as she walks behind the shooting lines will use the cues and 7 steps on a check off sheet. The individual final shooting scores could also be recorded, including scores from each distance.

Application To Golf:

This lesson can be applied to golf. The learning focus could be the full golf swing, chipping or putting. The instructional cues would be broken down very specifically on a reciprocal sheet for the partner to monitor. Whiffle golf balls could be used in the beginning and then depending on the class and space, regulation golf balls. The students could practice hitting for "targets" such as hula-hoops, archery targets, laundry baskets or other creative ideas for targets. Practice activities could be set up in a similar way and the culminating activity would be a series of challenging stations set up as a mini golf course. The assessment would be the peer and teacher observation check off sheet.

Instructional Cues For Partner

STANCE	Straddle shooting line Weight evenly distributed Feet shoulder width apart
NOCK	Bow at side, string side up, inside arm Notch in the arrow just above horizontal Bring fingers up from under, using index and next 2 fingers Use 1st joint of those 3 fingers, thumb up, little finger down.
DRAW	Bow arm is elbow out (do not roll in) Bow shoulder does not lift Squeeze shoulder blades together Flat, not cupped hand, string pressure even Fingers and arms are a hook (with no power)
ANCHOR	String bisects face (center of chin and nose) Index finger under jaw, thumb toward ear
AIM	Close correct eye Align string with eye
RELEASE	Open or straighten fingers, hand pulls back slightly Keep fingers in contact with neck
FOLLOW THROUGH	Hold and freeze "Pose for a picture" Take time to think about the shot

Assessment Check Sheet

Student Name: _____

Directions: The partner calls off the main heading and the shooter slowly and carefully goes through each of the cues in that step. The partner puts a + if they perform the specific movement and a − if they do not.

STANCE

_____ Straddle line

_____ Feet shoulder width apart

NOCK

_____ Arrow notched above horizontal

_____ 3 middle fingers at the 1st joint

DRAW

_____ Elbow out

_____ Shoulder down

ANCHOR

_____ String bisects face

_____ Finger under jaw, thumb on ear

AIM

_____ Close eye

RELEASE

_____ Throw fingers open

_____ Thumb and index finger stay on neck

FOLLOW THROUGH

_____ Hold and freeze

Resources

Published by the National Association for Sport and Physical Education for quality physical education programs:

Moving Into the Future: National Standards for Physical Education, A Guide to Content and Assessment (1995), Stock No. 304-10083

Concepts and Principles of Physical Education: What Every Student Needs to Know (2003), Stock No. 304-10261

Beyond Activities: Elementary Volume (2003), Stock No. 304-10265

Beyond Activities: Secondary Volume (2003), Stock No. 304-10268

National Physical Education Standards in Action (2003), 304-10267

Active Start: A Statement of Physical Activity Guidelines for Children Birth to Five Years (2002), Stock No. 304-10254

Physical Activity for Children: A Statement of Guidelines (1998), Stock No. 304-10175

National Standards for Beginning Physical Education Teachers (1995), Stock No. 304-10085

Appropriate Practice Documents

Appropriate Practice in Movement Programs for Young Children, (2000), Stock No. 304-10232

Appropriate Practices for Elementary School Physical Education (2000), Stock No. 304-10230

Appropriate Practices for Middle School Physical Education (2001), Stock No. 304-10248

Appropriate Practices for High School Physical Education (1998), Stock No. 304-10129

Opportunity to Learn Documents

Opportunity to Learn Standards for Elementary Physical Education (2000), Stock No. 304-10242

Physical Education Program Improvement and Self-Study Guides (1998) *for Middle School*, Stock No. 304-10173, *for High School*, Stock No. 304-10174

Assessment Series

Assessment in Outdoor Adventure Physical Education (2003),
Stock No. 304-10218

Assessing Student Outcomes in Sport Education (2003), Stock No. 304-10219

Video Tools for Teaching Motor Skill Assessment (2002), Stock No. 304-10217

Assessing Heart Rate in Physical Education (2002), Stock No. 304-10214

Authentic Assessment of Physical Activity for High School Students (2002),
Stock No. 304-10216

Portfolio Assessment for K-12 Physical Education (2000), Stock No. 304-10213

Elementary Heart Health: Lessons and Assessment (2001), Stock No. 304-10215

Standards-Based Assessment of Student Learning: A Comprehensive Approach
(1999), Stock No. 304-10206

Assessment in Games Teaching (1999), Stock No. 304-10212

Assessing Motor Skills in Elementary Physical Education (1999),
Stock No. 304-10207

Assessing and Improving Fitness in Elementary Physical Education (1999),
Stock No. 304-10208

Creating Rubrics for Physical Education (1999), Stock No. 304-10209

Assessing Student Responsibility and Teamwork (1999), Stock No. 304-10210

Preservice Professional Portfolio System (1999), Stock No. 304-10211

Order online at **www.aahperd.org/naspe** or call **1-800-321-0789**

Shipping and handling additional.

 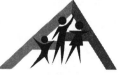

National Association for
Sport and Physical Education

an association of the American Alliance for Health,
Physical Education, Recreation and Dance

1900 Association Drive
Reston, VA 20191
(703) 476-3410
www.aahperd.org/naspe